YOU WANT TO TAKE
BODY . . . AND EXCEL IN
MUSCLE HWLCSC ANCING
MIRACLE YOU'VE BEEN LOOKING FOR?

THIS EXPERT GUIDE TAKES THE CONFUSION
AND FRUSTRATION OUT OF DECIDING WHAT'S
BEST FOR YOU, YOUR BODY, AND YOUR
SPORTS PERFORMANCE!

*Can creatine be taken with other supplements?
*What are the additional health benefits of creatine
and other supplements?
*How much is enough and
when should you stop?
*Should parents of young athletes . . .   rs

*Are all supplements . . . the same?
*Can women benefit from creatine?
*How can muscle boosters maximize a total sports
enhancement program?

FIND THESE ANSWERS AND MORE IN . . .

CREATINE AND OTHER
NATURAL MUSCLE BOOSTERS

PLUS: actual case histories that show what muscle
boosters can and can't do for you . . . common
questions and concerns . . . how to get the most
out of a workout program . . . and more!

CREATINE

AND OTHER

NATURAL

MUSCLE

BOOSTERS

Robert Monaco, M.D.
AND Terry Malloy

A Dell Book

Published by
Dell Publishing
a division of
Random House, Inc.
1540 Broadway
New York, New York 10036

Cover design by Melody Cassen

Dell books may be purchased for business or promotional use or for special sales. For information please write to: Special Markets Department, Random House, Inc., 1540 Broadway, New York, NY 10036.

Dell® is a registered trademark of Random House, Inc., and the colophon is a trademark of Random House, Inc.

ISBN: 0-440-23555-3

Printed in the United States of America

Published simultaneously in Canada

December 1999

10 9 8 7 6 5 4 3 2

OPM

Robert Monaco, M.D., would
like to give special thanks to the
following individuals for their
patience, support, and assistance
in the book: cm, bch, tg, mk, cm, em,
jm, dc, and cz.

Contents

Note to Readers

The material in this book is for informational purposes only. It is not intended to serve as a prescription manual, or to replace the advice and care of your medical doctor. Although every effort has been made to provide the most up-to-date information, the medical science in this field and the information about creatine and other natural muscle boosters are rapidly changing. Therefore, we strongly recommend that you consult with your doctor before using any of the drugs or supplements discussed in this book. The authors and publisher expressly disclaim responsibility for any adverse effects that may result from the use or application of the information contained in this book.

Introduction

Suddenly, it was front-page news. Creatine builds muscles. Creatine improves strength. Creatine delays fatigue. Creatine measurably enhances athletic performance.

And from everything known so far creatine is also very safe.

Does it all sound too good to be true? Can a powdery supplement from the health-food store really make such a difference? The resounding answer for many is yes!

If you're thin and want to bulk up, if you're big and want to muscle up, or if you're just looking for better performance in your sport or exercise routine, creatine may well be the boost you've been searching for.

Since its commercial introduction in 1993 annual sales of this nutritional supplement have skyrocketed. Whether it's in powder form or in tablets, capsules, liquids, gels, chewable wafers, gum, or even candy, sports enthusiasts can't get enough of it. Creatine is literally flying off the shelves. In fact, it's by far America's best-selling strength and energy supplement.

The media tell us that pro athletes like Dallas Cowboy Troy Aikman, Chicago Cub Sammy Sosa, and Olympic sprinter Michael Johnson are using it. In fact, estimates are that as many as half of all professional football players and at least one quarter of professional baseball players are taking creatine. Probably more. And the numbers are growing.

Maybe this supplement is not for everyone and maybe it does not work every single time. But for a large number of physically active people, creatine can help make the difference between winning and losing.

MARK MCGWIRE'S REVELATIONS

It all started innocently enough. It was near the end of August 1998. A bunch of reporters were gathered around the locker of Mark McGwire, the six-foot-five-inch, 250-pound St. Louis Cardinals slugger who was on the road to making baseball history for most home runs in a season.

Suddenly, a reporter noticed something in McGwire's locker, something that was in plain view: a bottle of the controversial muscle-enhancing supplement androstenedione.

What was this, anyway? Was McGwire's athletic superiority nothing more than the result of a pill? Were other players taking this stuff? What else were McGwire and other professional athletes ingesting to enhance their abilities?

And if McGwire broke the home-run record, would they have to put an asterisk next to his name to let everyone know he was only able to do it with the aid of a controversial supplement? That he couldn't do it fair and square? That he had to cheat?

Within hours the open secret known to many pro athletes, and to amateurs as well, was suddenly front-page news. Now everyone in the world had wised up. And the message was this: To make it in sports you need more than natural ability and hard work. You need a chemical boost.

McGwire protested that his use of androstenedione (known as "andro") was perfectly legal. In fact, although andro had been banned by the NCAA (National Collegiate Athletic Association), the National Football League, and the Olympics, it was permitted in baseball. Even so, as we will see, it is a very controversial and potentially dangerous substance.

But McGwire was also taking a second supplement, one that has been widely tested, apparently builds muscle effectively, and seems to have very few side effects: creatine.

The publicity resulting from McGwire's revelations dramatically increased public awareness that:

• A vast number of athletes, professional and amateur, male and female, teenager to senior citizen, are using nutritional supplements to strengthen muscles and improve performance.

• Some of these substances are safe and some are not.

- Some of these substances are effective and some are not.

- Some of these supplements have been widely tested and some have not.

- In addition, many athletes use illegal drugs to enhance performance, and these can have serious health effects (even including death), result in records being overturned, and end in suspension or even permanent banning from their sports.

- Of all the supplements available to enhance muscular strength, the most widely used and most effective, according to research, is creatine.

QUESTIONS ABOUT CREATINE AND OTHER SUPPLEMENTS

There are many questions to answer. For example, which creatine product is the best? Or are they all basically about the same? Does each one contain the same amount of creatine? What about other ingredients that may be included in the product? Are they necessary and do they help build muscle?

How much should I take? How often should I take it? Should I take it alone or with meals? What's the best liquid to mix it with? Should I load up when I first start taking it? Should I cycle, that is, take it for a while and then take a break from it? If I'm young and still growing, could it be dangerous to my natural growth?

This book will answer all these questions and more. It will tell you the story of creatine, how it was discovered, how it acts in your body, and how you can use it effectively to build muscles and enhance your athletic performance.

But you need to know more than just how good creatine can be. We will also alert you to a variety of possible side effects and dangers, and let you know who should and who should not be using creatine supplements.

You will also learn that creatine is not effective in every sport, and in some sports it may actually hurt your performance. It's important to know this before you start using it.

Like that of any nutritional supplement the story of creatine is complicated. If you're reading this book, the chances are you want to take good care of your body and you also want to excel in sports, two goals that go hand in hand. Supplements can sometimes help, but you need to know what you're doing before you use them.

Don't be swayed because all your friends are using certain supplements, or because Mark McGwire or other famous and successful pros are taking them.

Don't think that the only road to victory in sports is through taking expensive and popular formulas that may be a waste of your money or even hazardous to your health.

To help you find the answers this book will discuss creatine at length, as well as some of the other supplements sports enthusiasts are using to build muscle, including andro, whey protein, glutamine, DHEA, steroids, HMB, pyruvate, chromium, and GBL.

By examining the facts and applying them to your specific situation, you will be able to make intelligent and informed choices about supplement use and figure out what will work best for you, your body, your overall health, and your sports performance.

Chapter 1

Nutritional Supplements and the Competitive Edge

WHY CREATINE?

There are many reasons why creatine has emerged as the clear winner in the sports nutritional supplement arena. Creatine has been shown to:

- increase muscle mass (size)
- boost muscle strength
- possibly speed the rate of muscle growth
- possibly prevent breakdown of muscle tissue
- help the body lose fat and replace it with lean muscle
- increase the body's production of adenosine triphosphate (ATP), the fuel used for fast bursts of activity
- shorten recovery time during activities (such as between reps) and between workouts
- possibly delay muscle fatigue
- permit longer and more intense workouts
- improve athletic performance, especially when

short bursts of strength are required, as in power lifting, bodybuilding, wrestling, sprinting, martial arts, football, baseball, hockey, javelin, discus, shot put, hammer throwing, and other sports

- possibly elevate levels of HDL (the good kind of) cholesterol
- help improve body image
- possibly increase motivation to train hard
- as of this writing, be safe, for short-term use, with few side effects
- possibly have benefits in treating certain medical conditions, including Lou Gehrig's disease, congestive heart failure, recovery from surgery, AIDS-related muscular wasting, and loss of muscular strength in the elderly
- help in about 80 percent of the people who try it

On the downside you should note that creatine:

- should not be used by people with kidney problems
- may not help endurance athletes in such sports as long-distance running or swimming, and may even be a negative factor, since its use can result in weight gain
- may have side effects such as cramping, nausea, and diarrhea in some people who use it
- may cause dehydration by drawing water into the muscle cells

- may have no noticeable effect on sports performance for some people, possibly those who already have high levels of creatine in their muscles
- may do little or nothing unless you exercise on a regular basis while taking it
- may be dangerous if taken in larger-than-recommended doses
- has no long-term studies to prove there are no adverse side effects when used over a period of years

THE SEARCH FOR A BOOST

We've all seen them. People wandering around health-food stores, picking up one product after another, reading labels and considering: *will this work for me or not?* They talk to the clerks, compare ingredients, and try to choose the right supplement, the one that will be worth the money and make a difference in their performance, make them stronger and more energetic.

Chances are, you've done this yourself, so you know the feeling.

It's confusing. And frustrating. There are so many products, so many different manufacturers, such a variety of formulas. One promises "high energy," another says it will "fuel muscles," while yet another claims their product will "enable the muscles to work at greater intensity."

How can you know if these claims are true? Do you need to be a chemist or physician or nutritionist to be able to figure it out? And are there any governmental safeguards, or can these manufacturers just make any claim they want to? These are some of the things you should know before buying.

If you walk into a health-food store today, things look very different from a few years ago. Now, instead of row after row of vitamin and mineral bottles, chances are the first thing you'll see as you come in the door is a big selection of creatine products.

Creatine seems to be everywhere. The figure of $200 million in annual sales makes a pretty important statement. People want this stuff and they're willing to pay for it. Thirty, forty, even fifty dollars a month and sometimes more. Is it really worth it?

SUPPLEMENT REGULATIONS

We all know that prescription medications are carefully regulated by the FDA (Food and Drug Administration), and drug manufacturers spend millions of dollars researching their products to prove they are safe and effective, so they can gain FDA approval and sell them to the public. In fact, recent statistics indicate that some drug manufacturers spend up to $500 million on developing a single drug.

But what about nutritional supplements?

Manufacturers of dietary supplements have an estimated annual revenue of $11.5 billion dollars. It seems like just about everyone takes at least one multivitamin per day, and millions of people take a whole menu of products, including individual vitamin and mineral pills, herbal remedies, and protein supplements.

But since these supplements are neither drugs nor food, the FDA has no power to regulate them.

For years a great battle has been waged between the government and the public over the question of regulations. Health-food advocates claim it is their right to take any nutritional supplements they want and the government has no business interfering. "We can self-regulate," they argue, "and we don't want the government telling us what we can and can't take for our health." Government officials counter that there must be strict controls if the public safety is to be assured.

The Dietary Supplement and Health Education Act of 1994 grew out of this debate. It allows manufacturers to produce and sell nutritional supplements, provided they are not considered drugs by the FDA and companies make no health or medical claims for their products. Creatine, andro, and all the other supplements you buy in the health-food store come under this act. In addition, these nutritional supplements do not have to be clinically tested for effectiveness or safety.

However, there are exceptions. If the FTC (Federal Trade Commission) finds that a producer is using misleading advertising or making claims it cannot substantiate, this government agency can take legal action against the manufacturer in order to protect the public.

In addition, the FDA can take action against supplement manufacturers whose products cause serious health risks to their users. This was the case in 1989, when the amino acid supplement L-tryptophan caused about thirty-eight deaths, apparently due to accidental contamination in a Japanese factory. As a result the FDA banned tryptophan for sale in this country.

So despite the power of these agencies, at this time there is really very little government control over the content of dietary supplements. Quality can widely vary from product to product, and the motto is "buyer beware."

However, there is some hope on the horizon for the consumer. In a regulation that went into effect in early 1999, the FDA now requires manufacturers of dietary supplements to provide more complete information on their labels.

Specifically, they must include a complete list of all ingredients and the precise levels of every vitamin, mineral, herb, or other substance in the product, similar to what is provided for most food items in the supermarket.

With this new "supplement facts" label, people who buy creatine and other supplements will have a better chance to judge each product and make an informed decision about what to buy. They will be able to see, quickly and easily, exactly what ingredients the product contains and in what amounts. As a result, comparison shopping should be much less confusing.

THE PURSUIT OF VICTORY

Let's face it. There's nothing like winning.

In a split second you feel an intoxicating rush unlike anything else you will ever know.

The quest for this singular thrill is what motivates many athletes around the world. Whether you're a twelve-year-old figure skater getting up at five in the morning to train for the Olympics, a basketball player shooting hoops all weekend, or a runner snatching a few extra laps in the cold winter dark after work, you are willing to go the extra mile, push your body to the limit, in fact, do almost anything just to gain that infinitesimal competitive edge that can be the difference between second place and first. Between almost making it and breaking a record. Between winning and losing.

Throughout history athletes have trained to perfect their bodies and their performance, running, jumping, lifting weights, whether at home alone, on school teams, in neighborhood playgrounds, in gyms, or in professional sports. And until recently the ingredients that made up a good athlete were pretty simple: natural ability, hard work, good health, and the will to succeed.

But now the formula has changed. There's been a significant addition, a new factor that can actually alter the balance: supplements.

Everyone's doing it, right?

Before you join the crowds take a moment to inform yourself. Or if you're already taking supplements, do yourself a favor and find out more about them. *And above all, do not take any supplements, no matter how safe you may think they are, without a doctor's approval and supervision.*

In today's world you have to be alert. You have to be smart. You have to know what you're doing. As the saying goes, you've got to look out for number one—it's not such bad advice.

So if you're just starting an exercise program for the

first time, or if you want to maintain and enhance your regular fitness program, or if you're a serious athlete and want to dramatically improve your performance, you should know more about creatine. It could be the answer to your prayers.

Chapter 2

What Is Creatine?

Creatine is not just a powdered supplement that you buy, mix up, and swallow. It's also already in your body, a natural and important substance found mainly in the muscles of humans and most animals.

Creatine is made up of three amino acids: arginine, glycine, and methionine. Some people call it an amino acid, others a protein, and others a nutrient. Scientifically, it's an "N-methyl-guanidinoacetic acid," or a "crystallizable nitrogenous compound synthesized in the body."

Creatine's main job is to fuel energy in the muscles, especially for the rapid and intense bursts we often need in sports. It does this in the form of creatine phosphate (or phosphocreatine) in our muscle cells.

About 95 percent of the creatine in our bodies is found in the skeletal muscles, with the remainder in other areas of the body, including the heart, brain, testes, retina, and other tissues.

The average man has about 120 grams (or 4 ounces)

of creatine in his body, with about 95 percent in skeletal muscles.

Creatine has been called an important "ergogenic" aid, which means it is effective in increasing work output, or energy, which is so vital in sports, exercise, and other intense activities.

SOURCES OF CREATINE

Although creatine is concentrated in the muscles, it isn't made there. Instead, 1 to 2 grams of creatine are produced each day in our liver, kidneys, and pancreas. The body also obtains creatine directly from the food we eat, mainly meat, fish, and animal products. The creatine is transported through the bloodstream into the muscles.

So the body has two main sources of creatine:

- creatine made in the body from amino acids, and stored in the muscles, and
- creatine obtained directly from the diet, especially meat and fish

Creatine is made primarily from three amino acids:

- *arginine,* a conditionally essential amino acid that is responsible for the release of growth hormone and is important in the healing of wounds
- *glycine,* a nonessential amino acid that stimulates the release of growth hormone, and
- *methionine,* an essential amino acid that helps to prevent fat concentration in the liver and acts as an antioxidant

Amino Acids

Known as the "building blocks of life," amino acids are the substances that make up proteins in the tissues of all living organisms. Twenty-three in number, they are vital for the body to grow, maintain, and repair itself.

Inside the body various amino acids combine in different ways to form an endless number of different types of protein. Thirteen of these amino acids can be manufactured by the body, but the other nine cannot and require ingredients from the food you eat.

Essential amino acids are the ones needed for protein synthesis that our bodies cannot make and must obtain from our diet.

Nonessential amino acids are the ones needed for protein synthesis that our bodies can make, and they are not specifically required in the diet.

Conditionally essential amino acids are in between and are partially made in the body and partially dependent on dietary sources. They are needed from food under certain conditions, such as extreme stress, when the body's stores become depleted and additional supplies must be provided by the diet.

Once the organs have taken these three amino acids and manufactured creatine, it travels through the bloodstream to the muscles. The creatine is stored in our muscle cells until it is needed for the energy we use to move when we make muscle contractions.

Finally, our bodies also convert 1 to 2 grams of creatine into creatinine each day, which then passes through the kidneys and is excreted in urine.

DIETARY CREATINE AND ITS USE

The average person eats about 1 or 2 grams of creatine a day, but people who eat large amounts of meat, fish, or animal products take in more. Because of this and other factors, each of us has a different amount of creatine in the muscles. Strict vegetarians have less because they are not eating meat, fish, or animal products, such as milk or cheese. But the body does compensate slightly to attempt to maintain normal levels.

There are also genetic, physiological differences among people, and each person has a different amount of creatine in his or her body at any given time. Men, for instance, may have more stored creatine than women.

In order to maintain normal body metabolism the average person uses about 2 grams of creatine a day. For some people this is more than they take in through their food. So for those who are very physically active their dietary source of creatine may not be adequate over a period of time.

Repetitive intense exercise depletes creatine stores at their local muscle sites. As physical exertion continues day after day, these creatine stores may decrease and people will experience muscle fatigue and the inability to do high-intensity work as effectively as they would like.

Therefore, many of these very active people may benefit from taking creatine supplements, which are sold in the form of creatine monohydrate. This is especially true of people who engage in sports requiring short-term (ten- to thirty-second) spurts of energy, which require large amounts of creatine.

By using supplemental creatine sports enthusiasts

find that their muscles can quickly rebuild stores of energy, allowing them to train and play harder and longer, and with less fatigue.

By adding creatine supplements to your regimen you provide your body with an important third way to obtain this essential nutrient.

Before we look at exactly the way in which creatine builds muscle and strength in the body, we need to understand exactly how our muscles operate.

CREATINE CONTENT OF SOME FOODS

Food	Creatine Content (grams per pound)
Herring	3.0
Pork	2.3
Beef	2.0
Salmon	2.0
Tuna	1.8
Codfish	1.4
Milk	0.05

Note: Theoretically, you can increase your creatine levels and your athletic performance through diet modifications, by eating foods that are high in creatine. However, you would have to eat something like four to eight steaks a day in order to get the amounts of creatine that you need to see performance enhancement. Also, these foods can be high in fat and have excess calories that you may not want.

Chapter 3

How Muscles Work

We all want big, hard, strong muscles, but we need to build them slowly and safely. It's easy to get obsessed with your body and to want fast results so badly that you do things you might regret later on.

To understand how to build your muscles in a safe, effective, and long-lasting way, it's a good idea to first understand how they work. The process is a little complicated, but once you get the idea, you'll be able to make the best choices to attain maximum growth.

WHAT ARE MUSCLES?

Muscles are what allow your body to move. Without them you would not be able to walk, open your eyes, eat, or breathe. In fact, your blood would stop circulating, your heart would stop beating, and you would simply die.

A muscle is an organ that produces movement by means of contraction (becoming shorter and thicker). Muscles almost always appear in pairs, one to perform the contraction and one to assist it back to the original position. More than six hundred muscles are found throughout the body.

DIFFERENT TYPES OF MUSCLE

The body has three main types of muscle: skeletal or striated, smooth, and cardiac. They work in a similar way, but each does a different job.

Skeletal or striated muscles are attached to the bones throughout your body, and it is their action that moves your bones.

Smooth muscles are found in the blood vessels, stomach, intestines, glands, and skin, and keep these body parts working properly.

Cardiac muscle is found only in the heart and is responsible for the heart continually pumping blood to keep you alive.

The muscles in the body are classified as voluntary and involuntary.

Voluntary muscles, including the skeletal muscles, act in response to a message from the brain. In other words they act when you want them to, whether it's to walk to the mailbox, bend to pick up a box, or chew your food. When they get the message to move, they shorten, pulling one bone toward the other. Then, for example, you can bend your arm or your leg. This happens when one of the muscle pair contracts. Then, when you want your arm or leg to unbend, the other muscle in the pair relaxes it back into place.

Involuntary muscles, like smooth and cardiac muscles, act without any direct messages from the brain.

They carry on their work automatically in order to keep the organs and glands in your body working on their own and so keep you alive without your having to think about it all the time.

SOME MUSCLES USED IN EXERCISE

Since there are over six hundred muscles in the body, most people aren't familiar with all of them. But for those who are involved in sports, certain muscles keep coming up over and over.

Biceps and triceps: Found in the upper arm, these muscles are long and wiry in shape. They work together to bend the elbows and allow movement in the fore-arms. When you want to bend your arm, the biceps contract; when you want to straighten it out, the triceps contract to pull your arm back into its original straight position.

Brachioradialis, supinator, and pronator teres: These muscles are located in the forearm and work together to allow movement in the wrists and hands.

Pectoralis major and pectoralis minor: Located on both sides of the chest, these muscles are composed of flat bands of tissue that act to move the shoulders and the upper arms.

Trapezius, teres major, teres minor, deltoid, and latissimus dorsi: These muscles are located in the back and are involved in movements of the back, arms, shoulders, and neck.

Gluteus maximus, gluteus medius, and gluteus minimus: Located in the lower rear of the torso, these muscles are responsible for movements in the hips and are involved in such activities as sitting, bending, running, and climbing.

Quadriceps: These muscles are found in the upper leg and are essential for straightening your leg and assisting you when you are running or walking.

Soleus and gastrocnemius: Found in the lower leg or calf, these muscles help you move your ankles and feet and help maintain balance so you can walk, run, and jump.

INJURIES

When someone has an injury, the muscles may be affected. When you strain muscles by working them too hard to the point where they can't do the job, you may experience a muscle strain or sprain. You will experience pain, which can be intense, and difficulty in movement. Of course, the injury will have to be treated. Eventually, with rest and recuperation, the muscle usually repairs itself.

However, if you have been forced to avoid exercise while you are recuperating, you will find that when you first begin to use your injured limb again, it will be very weak. The lack of use has debilitated the muscles and it will take some time for them to get back the strength they had before you were injured.

Far more serious are various types of brain injuries, which can sometimes make it difficult or even impossible for someone to direct the voluntary muscles to work. In addition, spinal-cord injuries can sever the nerves that carry messages from the brain, and cause the same result. So even though the brain is working perfectly well, the message can't get through and the muscles do not move the body part the brain tells them to move. This condition, paralysis, comes in varying degrees and locations, and may be temporary or permanent.

WHAT MUSCLES NEED

In order to grow, muscles need food and oxygen. And naturally, the more they are used, the more food and oxygen they will need.

We all know this from experience. When you were a young child learning to play basketball, for example, chances are you couldn't keep up with the older children or your parents. Your body was too small and your muscles too undeveloped, and before long you found you were out of breath and your body was aching from the strain.

But as you grew and used your muscles, they developed. If you are an adult and have been physically active all your life, your muscles will be more developed and you will be able to do more physical work than someone your age who has been sedentary and not used his or her muscles as much.

But let's move to the next step. Let's say you're mature, healthy, active, and able to do a lot, but you still want more.

Maybe you're a bodybuilder and want to tone and define your muscles. Maybe you're into sports and want to win a wrestling championship. Maybe you have your eye on eventually becoming a black belt in karate. Or maybe you're just getting older and don't have the same strength you did a few years ago. Whatever it is, you're always pushing your muscles to the max and you know you need an extra boost.

So the question arises: how can you get your muscles to be even bigger and do even more?

HOW MUSCLES GROW: HYPERTROPHY

The process by which muscles grow in size or mass is called "hypertrophy." Basically, it works like this:

As you work out and use your muscles, there are very small, minute tears in the muscle. In other words, the muscles are being damaged. It sounds like something bad, but what happens next is that the body moves to repair these tears, and in the process the muscles regrow and become bigger and stronger.

But this will only occur if the damage is not too great and if the body is given time to rest while the rebuilding takes place. That's why it may not be a good idea to work out seven days a week, or at least not do the same types of activities every single day.

For the weekend warrior this usually isn't a big problem. But for the dedicated exercise or sports enthusiast who can't miss a day, it might be. It could lead to slower growth or even injuries, as the muscles are damaged over and over before they have the chance to repair.

So, in order to maximize muscle growth, you have to know what you're doing. You have to exercise right and eat right. And if you choose to, you also have to supplement right.

Chapter 4

The History of Creatine

With all the excitement over creatine you'd think it has just recently been discovered. But the truth is, creatine was first discovered way back in 1832 by the French organic chemist Michel-Eugène Chevreul. Chevreul, famous for his research on fats, was also the first to identify various fatty acids such as oleic acid, butyric acid, and capric acid. He named his new discovery "creatine" after the Greek word for "flesh."

Creatine was first discovered in meat, and in 1847 scientists realized there was a greater concentration of creatine in the muscles of foxes killed in the wild than there was in the muscles of domesticated foxes. Their conclusion? Activity causes creatine to build up in the muscles.

Then in 1926 an article in a British medical journal said that creatine in its natural form can help people gain weight. By then it was known that the total amount of creatine stored in the average person's body was about 100 grams.

Scientists continued to study creatine, discovering that it is stored in muscles throughout the body, and eating creatine-rich food can add to the body's stores.

Looking to increase the body's supplies of creatine beyond the relatively small amounts that you can get from your food, scientists first developed synthetic creatine in the late 1950s. Made in America by Pfanstiehl Laboratories, an Illinois pharmaceutical company, the simple formula involved combining, and heating water with, two salts, cyanamide and sarcosine.

Before long, word got out that using this supplement could improve athletic performance. By the late 1960s or early 1970s many of the Eastern bloc countries were using synthetic creatine, along with dangerous anabolic steroids, in order to build up the strength and stamina of their athletes.

By the 1980s scientists had learned that muscles could be "loaded up" with creatine through the use of supplementation and that muscle stores could be increased by as much as 30 percent.

Then, during the 1992 Summer Olympics, the news media found out that several medal winners were supplementing with creatine, including British sprinters Linford Christie and Colin Jackson.

Finally, in 1993, creatine became available as a nutritional supplement in the American market. But even before that, some American athletes looking for extra support were taking it, including Baltimore Orioles center fielder Brady Anderson, who says he first used creatine in 1991.

But while studies and anecdotal evidence have cast

dark shadows over anabolic steroids, andro, and some other muscle-enhancing substances, the reputation of creatine has remained rather pristine. To date it is one of the more studied dietary supplements, and so far the results look pretty good.

SCIENTIFIC STUDIES

Estimates of the number of scientific studies on creatine are as high as two hundred. And the studies continue.

Some of these studies have yielded important information on how creatine works in the body, especially in regard to intense physical activities, including many sports. But there has also been some criticism about the meaning of the evidence because:

- few studies have measured creatine use for more than three months
- there are no long-term studies that follow creatine use over a period of years
- many studies were paid for by supplement manufacturers
- many studies used different protocols and therefore cannot be compared to one another
- studies varied in rest-period protocols
- many studies used inadequate dose amounts to see effects
- some studies lacked muscle biopsies
- most studies did not use sport-specific tasks
- studies failed to control for the effect of weight gain on performance

- many studies with positive results used trained athletes, so it is questionable that all the positive results were due to creatine use alone

Therefore, we have to be very careful when we evaluate all the evidence. And we cannot believe or base all our decisions on one study alone. But if a study is well designed and its results are repeated by multiple independent labs, we may conclude that we have accurate results.

Even so, there are still a large number of studies, done in the United States and in other countries, that indicate creatine is safe and effective in helping to build muscle. We will look at some of the more significant studies.

PERFORMANCE BENEFIT STUDIES

The 1992 Harris Study

Creatine researchers consider this study the pioneering research on creatine. It was conducted by Roger Harris and his associates in the laboratory of Dr. Eric Hultman at the Karolinska Institute in Stockholm, Sweden, in the late 1980s and was published in a scientific journal (*Clinical Science*) in 1992, under the title "Elevation of creatine in resting and exercised muscles of normal subjects by creatine supplementation."

The Harris study was designed to find out if the use of creatine supplements would increase the levels of creatine in the muscles and the blood. The study's findings showed that levels of creatine in the muscles could be increased up to 50 percent with the use of creatine supplementation.

The researchers used seventeen volunteers who were given 5 grams of creatine monohydrate every day. The creatine, mixed with hot tea or coffee, was taken either four or six times per day for two or more days. The results were an increase in the creatine contents of every subject's muscles, with the volunteers having the lowest concentrations before supplementation showing the greatest gain (as high as 50 percent).

The researchers found that the first two days of supplementation resulted in the greatest gain of creatine stores in the thigh muscles (quadriceps femoris), which averaged about 32 percent. They also tested their subjects by having them exercise only one leg and found that the exercised leg elevated creatine stores by about 37 percent while the nonexercised leg's creatine stores increased by just 25 percent.

Here are the conclusions from that study:

• Creatine stores in the muscles can be increased by supplementation.
• The greatest increase comes in the first two days of supplementation (a conclusion that led to the concept of creatine loading, which will be explained later).
• Physical activity increases creatine stores.

The 1993 Greenhaff Study

The next important creatine study was also conducted in Sweden at the Karolinska Institute, this time by Paul Greenhaff and his colleagues, including Dr. Eric Hultman. It was published in the same journal, *Clinical Science,* in 1993 under the title "Influence of oral creatine supplementation on muscle torque during repeated bouts of maximal voluntary exercise in man."

What Greenhaff and his associates looked at in this study was whether or not creatine supplementation was beneficial for intense physical activity. Using twelve volunteers, a small number, the researchers divided the group and gave half a creatine monohydrate supplement of 5 grams a day (mixed with 1 gram of glucose in hot tea or coffee) and the other half a placebo of 6 grams of glucose. Of course, neither group knew whether they were receiving the creatine or the placebo.

(A placebo, often used in scientific research, is an inactive medicine that looks like the real medicine and is usually given to one half of the test subjects. Then, at the end of the study, the group that is taking the placebo is compared to the group that is taking the real medicine and the differences are noted.)

The volunteers were asked to exercise before they were given the supplements (or placebo) and then again five days after taking the supplements (or placebo). The results of their exercise were then measured to determine whether the use of supplementary creatine has an effect on physical activity.

The specific exercise done by the subjects was five rounds of thirty leg extension-contractions on an exercise machine, which were separated by one-minute recovery periods. Before and after these rounds the scientists measured the subjects' muscle torque production (torque is a measurement of stress or force by a source external to the body, which causes rotation) and their blood lactate and ammonia levels and looked for any differences.

What they found was that for the subjects taking the placebo, muscle peak torque production during exercise was the same before and after supplementation. But for the subjects taking creatine the muscle torque production was significantly greater toward the last few bouts of exercise.

This study is significant because normally, torque declines as exercise progresses because muscles get tired. Greenhaff and his associates showed that creatine could counteract this natural tendency and permit people who exercise to remain stronger for a longer period of time.

The 1993 Balsom Study

Once again this study was carried out in Hultman's laboratory in Sweden, this time by Paul Balsom and his colleagues, and published in *Scandinavian Journal of Medicine and Science in Sports,* under the title "Creatine supplementation and dynamic high-intensity intermittent exercise."

Here, Balsom and his associates wanted to study the influence of creatine supplements on high-intensity intermittent (discontinuous) exercise.

Their subjects were sixteen men, who were placed into two groups: those given 5 grams of creatine (with 1 gram of glucose) five times a day for six days and those given a placebo with the same frequency.

The exercise they were asked to perform was ten six-second rounds of high-speed cycling at two different intensities: 130 revolutions per minute and 140 revolutions per minute. These exercise sessions took place before and after supplementation.

The results were that the group on the placebo showed no difference in their results before or after they were given the supplement. The group on the creatine, however, showed better performances as they approached the end of the 140-rpm exercise.

The creatine group also showed a weight gain averaging 2.4 pounds after one month, while the placebo group showed none. The conclusions? Creatine appeared to account for improved performance in high-intensity exercise, especially toward the end of the brief spurts of activity. The reason? A greater concentration of creatine phosphate in the muscles of the group taking the creatine supplement and a quicker resynthesis rate of making creatine once it is used up.

The 1994 Birch Study

Here, coauthors R. Birch and D. Noble were joined by Paul Greenhaff, who has been involved in a number of creatine studies, many under his direction. Birch, Noble, and Greenhaff, scientists at the University of Nottingham Medical School in England, wanted to further test the effect of creatine supplementation on exercise performance and on accumulations of ammonia and lactic acid in the body.

The test subjects were fourteen men, some of whom were given 5 grams of creatine daily and others of whom were given a placebo. They were asked to exercise by doing three thirty-second rounds of rapid cycling, interspersed by four-minute rest periods before and after the supplementation.

The results published as "The influence of dietary creatine supplementation on performance during repeated bouts of maximal isokinetic cycling in man," in the *European Journal of Applied Physiology and Occupational Physiology,* showed that the group on the placebo showed no difference in performance. However, the group on creatine did 6 percent better in terms of energy on the first and second rounds of exercise; there was no measurable difference in the third round. There was also a lower accumulation of ammonia (a byproduct of fatigue), suggesting that the creatine worked by providing energy directly to the muscle. This indicates that creatine increases work output, at least for short-term intense exercise of the type performed.

The 1995 Earnest Study

The exercise used in this creatine study was weight lifting, the type of short-burst, intense exercise that seems to benefit from creatine supplementation. The study was conducted by C. P. Earnest and associates, representing Texas Women's University, the University of Texas Southwestern Medical Center, and the Cooper Clinic in Dallas. Presented at the 1994 annual meeting of the American College of Sports Medicine in Indianapolis, the study was published in *Acta Physiologica Scandinavica* in 1995 as "The effect of creatine monohydrate ingestion on anaerobic power indices, muscular strength, and body composition."

The study group consisted of eight weight-trained men who were divided into those given 5 grams of creatine four times a day, and those given a placebo. The men took the supplements for a period of twenty-eight days. Before and after taking the supplement the group were measured for their weight, body composition, and ability to perform repetitions of a bench press at maximal weight.

This study was important because it was the first to scientifically measure the effects of creatine supplements taken over a four-week period, longer than in previous studies.

The findings? Creatine produced significant increases in anaerobic capacity (not involving the presence of oxygen), while the placebo group showed no such increases. This meant that the men who took creatine were able to work harder and for a longer period of time, increasing their muscle growth. In addition, the men using creatine gained an average of 2 percent lean muscle mass within thirty days, an important demonstration of the effect of the supplement to increase muscle size.

The 1995 Balsom Study

Paul Balsom and associates in Sweden tested seven men with creatine supplements by having them perform rounds of exercise on a cycle ergometer, a device that measures the amount of work done by muscles. The men were given 20 grams of creatine a day for six days, a larger amount than many other studies. The study, published in 1995 in *Acta Physiologica Scandinavica*, was entitled "Skeletal muscle metabolism during short-duration high-intensity exercise: the influence of creatine supplementation."

The exercise performed consisted of five rounds of a six-second fixed-intensity workout, a thirty-second recovery period, then, after forty seconds, one ten-second maximal workout. Muscle extracts were taken from their legs in order to measure creatine content.

The findings were that creatine supplements had increased the amount of creatine stored in the muscles by an average of 20 percent at the point before the exercise began. After five rounds of exercise the muscular creatine content was far greater than it had been before the supplement was taken. The researchers also found that the creatine lessened the men's muscle fatigue and that there was an average weight gain of 2.4 pounds after six days of supplementation.

In a second part of the study ten-second maximum workouts were performed and the results showed that creatine increased work output by 5 percent.

An interesting finding was that no improvement was detected in the performance of jumps with creatine supplementation. This may be explained by the weight gain, which counteracted the ability to jump easily.

ADDITIONAL STUDIES

Many other studies have shown the positive effects of creatine on athletic performance. By having many other labs repeat the studies and show similar results, we can see that creatine does work. Proponents of quite a few other supplements refer to one or two studies that might show a benefit, but could not be reliably reproduced. Some of the additional studies on creatine include:

Prevost, 1997: Dr. Mike Prevost and associates at Louisiana State University showed that high-intensity activity lasting under ten seconds benefits from creatine supplementation. The test subjects were asked to use exercise bicycles and the ones on creatine did not seem to experience fatigue when the noncreatine subjects did, and said they felt they could continue exercising. The study was published as "Creatine supplementation enhances intermittent work performance," in *Research Quarterly for Exercise and Sport.*

Vandenberghe, 1997: This study, published as "Long-term creatine intake is beneficial to muscle performance during resistance training," in *The Journal of Applied Physiology,* studied young women who were involved in weight training. Those who took 20 grams of creatine for four days, then 5 grams of creatine for the following ten weeks, generated more strength and greater muscle development than the control group on the placebo.

McNaughton, 1998: L. R. McNaughton of Kingston University in England wanted to find out whether creatine supplementation would have a positive effect on performance using a kayak ergometer. Using sixteen test subjects, McNaughton and his associates gave one group creatine (5 grams four times a day for five days) and the other a placebo. They found that the group using creatine "completed significantly more work" than the placebo group and they concluded that "creatine supplementation can significantly increase the amount of work accomplished" during kayak ergometer testing.

The list of studies showing positive performance effects seems to go on and on. Richard Kreider, one of the leading researchers on creatine, summarized these studies in a recent article in the *Journal of Exercise Physiology On-line* at www.css.edu/users/tboone2.asep/jan3htm. He notes that creatine has been shown to improve the following:

- one repetition maximum and/or peak power
- vertical jump
- multiple sets of maximal effort muscle contraction
- single sprints lasting 6 to 30 seconds
- repetitive sprints (recovery 0.5–5 minutes)
- exercise lasting 1.5 to 5 minutes
- increased ventilatory anaerobic threshold (how long until you become fatigued)
- increased maximal exercise capacity

STUDIES SHOWING NEGATIVE EFFECTS

Not all creatine studies have shown benefits. But when you look at the science and physiology behind creatine (which we will discuss in greater detail later on), you cannot expect it to work all the time. No supplement can give you everything. So we will look at some of the studies showing creatine's failings. These studies can help us to understand exactly how creatine works and who should take it.

The 1994 Stroud Study

Again, at Nottingham, Michael Stroud and his co-researchers, including Paul Greenhaff, studied the effects of creatine on a steadier form of exercise, this time using a treadmill. Their paper was published in 1994 as "Effect of oral creatine supplementation on respiratory gas exchange and blood lactate accumulation during steady-state incremental treadmill exercise and recovery in man," in the journal *Clinical Science*.

The study group consisted of eight men who took 20 grams of creatine a day over a period of five days. The researchers then took a set of physical measurements on the men before and after activity, which consisted of seven sets of treadmill exercise, each lasting six minutes.

The findings were as follows: creatine was not found to have any significant effect on heart rate, oxygen consumption, blood-lactate concentration, respiratory exchange ratio, expired gas volume, or carbon dioxide production.

What does all that mean? It indicates that creatine may not be an effective energy-producing supplement when long-term, steady-state exercise is involved.

Other studies also showed that exercise lasting more than sixty seconds was not directly helped by creatine. These include articles by Godly on the effects of creatine on endurance cycling; Terrilon on the effects of creatine on two seven-hundred-meter maximal running bouts; Burke on the effects of creatine on single-effort sprint performance in elite swimmers; and Febbraio on the effects of creatine on intermittent, supramaximal exercise in humans.

Creatine also appears not to help sprints lasting six to sixty seconds when prolonged recovery periods are used (five to twenty-five minutes). This was noted by Burke in the above study on elite swimmers and confirmed by Mujika, who showed that creatine supplementation does not improve sprint performance in competitive sprinters. Cooke and Redondo showed similar results on the bike.

Kreider again summarized the types of exercise and/or exercise conditions in which creatine supplementation has been reported to provide no ergogenic benefits:

- exercise lasting more than sixty seconds, multiple studies
- repetitive sprints (recovery five to twenty-five minutes), multiple studies
- single sprints lasting six to thirty seconds, multiple studies

Single studies showed negative results for one repetition performed at maximum and/or peak force, work performed during low-intensity muscle contractions, and work performed during high-intensity muscle contractions. However, Kreider notes that many of these studies can be faulted, since they often did not use a high-enough dose (less than 20 g/day over the five-day load period), or control for other factors in their protocols that could have clearly affected the results.

So even with these negative studies the jury is still out on certain elements, like sprints. We do know, though, that creatine probably does not significantly affect endurance exercise.

LOADING STUDIES

The scientific studies also tell us about what might be the correct dose of creatine and where all that creatine you take is going. Some key studies are noted below.

The 1996 Greenhaff Studies

These two studies were published in journals, as "Carbohydrate ingestion augments skeletal muscle creatine accumulation during creatine supplementation in humans" (*American Journal of Physiology*) and "Carbohydrate ingestion augments creatine retention during creatine feeding in humans" (*Acta Physiologica Scandinavica*). The researchers, members of Greenhaff's group in England, wanted to study whether taking in a simple carbohydrate with creatine supplements increased the levels of creatine in the muscles, above those achieved by taking creatine alone.

The first study involved four groups of subjects: one took creatine alone, two groups took creatine plus a simple carbohydrate, and the last group took the placebo alone. One of the groups taking creatine and carbohydrate exercised on a daily basis. The findings were that adding a simple carbohydrate to creatine increased the body's retention of creatine and decreased creatine excretion. In this study there was no evidence that exercise increased creatine retention.

The second Greenhaff study involved taking samples from the muscles to test for creatine stores. The researchers found that the group receiving a simple carbohydrate with creatine had a 60 percent rise in creatine content in the muscles.

Note: Carbohydrates are substances found in food which are composed of carbon, hydrogen, and oxygen. They include starch, sugar, and cellulose and are the major components of most plants. Simple carbohydrates, such as glucose or dextrose, are sugars that the body can use directly, without further internal processing.

If other studies had used Greenhaff's protocol of administering creatine with a simple carbohydrate, such as that found in grape juice, they might have shown additional benefits for the supplement.

The Hultman Study

In 1996 Hultman published a study entitled "Muscle creatine loading in men," in *The Journal of Applied Physiology,* involving a study of thirty-one males. He noted that muscle creatine increased by approximately 20 percent after six days on 20 grams per day of creatine. Hultman also noted that similar benefits could be obtained by taking 3 grams per day over twenty-eight days. It just took a longer time for the creatine to reach the same levels in the muscle. As we will see, Hultman also noted that it took about twenty-eight days without creatine for the subjects to return to their normal levels of muscle creatine.

As mentioned earlier, Harris also found a similar loading phenomenon with creatine. Other researchers clearly substantiated these findings.

***

So when we look at all the loading studies on creatine, we can draw the following conclusions:

1. The typical loading dose of creatine should be 20 to 25 grams a day for five days.

2. Loading can increase total stores by 15 to 30 percent.

3. Using 3 grams of creatine daily for twenty-eight days without the loading phase will have similar effects to using the loading phase and then going on a maintenance dose.

4. Taking 0.3 g/kg of body weight daily for five days, followed by 0.03 g/kg daily as a maintenance dose may be another effective way of using creatine.

5. Carbohydrates taken with creatine may enhance creatine uptake in the muscles by as much as 10 to 20 percent.

6. The amount of creatine uptake is dependent on how much creatine you start with in your body.

7. Caffeine may block the absorption of creatine.

BODY COMPOSITION AND PHYSIOLOGY

The scientific studies on creatine also showed it to be of benefit for body composition. In addition, these studies helped to elucidate how creatine actually works.

The 1996 Kreider Studies

Richard B. Kreider, Ph.D., is one of the foremost creatine researchers in the field, has published many studies, and is continuing with his research into the effects of creatine on exercise. Director of the Exercise and Sport Nutrition Laboratory at the Human Movement Sciences and Education department of the University of Memphis in Tennessee, Dr. Kreider and his associates conducted two 1996 studies to assess the effects of creatine on the body during resistance training.

The first study, published in *Medicine and Science in Sports and Exercise* as "Effects of ingesting a lean-mass promoting supplement during resistance training on iso-kinetic performance," involved a group consisting of twenty-eight resistance-trained athletes who were studied over a twenty-eight-day period. They were divided into groups that were given either a low-calorie mixture with creatine, a high-calorie mixture with creatine, or carbohydrate powder alone (without creatine).

Researchers measured body composition before and after supplementation and found that the subjects taking creatine showed "a significantly greater increase in lean tissue weight, while fat weight was maintained."

In the second study, published in the *International Journal of Sports Medicine* in 1996 as "Effects of ingesting supplements designed to promote lean tissue accretion on body composition during resistance training," Kreider and his colleagues tried to duplicate the findings of the first study, but extended the test period to five weeks and used different supplement formulas.

The results were that at the end of the test period, the athletes on creatine had gained a greater amount of fat-free weight than the subjects who were not taking creatine. The researchers used creatine in two different doses, one higher and one lower. The subjects taking the higher creatine dose increased their fat-free weight by 7.6 pounds over the five-week period, while those on the lower-dose creatine increased their fat-free weight by only 5.4 pounds.

As mentioned earlier, Earnest and Balsom also showed similar responses. Other researchers (see Kreider's summary article) have confirmed these studies. In conclusion, these studies show that taking creatine supplements:

- increases creatine stores in the muscles
- enhances resynthesis of creatine
- does not affect oxygen uptake by the muscles and therefore does not affect aerobic activities
- increases lean fat-free mass may increase protein synthesis in muscle, thus increasing strength
- may enhance the effects of training on muscle hypertrophy
- may increase metabolic muscle efficiency

However, you should note that these studies may not be large enough to pick up subtle side effects.

SIDE-EFFECT STUDIES

There is far less scientific literature on side effects of creatine. This may be due to some reasons that we will explore in more detail later. These reasons might be:

- There are no significant side effects.
- We have not used creatine long enough to see any

significant side effects. Most studies only go out two years at most. But remember that creatine is a natural product in the body and that Europeans were using it as early as the 1960s and we have not, so far, heard of any serious problems.

- There are anecdotal reports of side effects (for example, cramping) but we do not yet have scientific proof showing that these are a result of creatine.

Because of this situation we should keep an eye on the evolving scientific literature on creatine and not simply accept the rumors or suppositions we may hear that have not been scientifically proven.

Mark Juhn, D.O., of the University of Washington performed a critical review of the potential side effects of oral creatine supplementation, which appeared in the *Clinical Journal of Sport Medicine*. Richard Kreider also reviewed the medical safety issues. In sum, they noted:

- Creatine does cause weight gain in many individuals. While this can be helpful to some, additional weight may hinder performance in specific sports, such as wrestling.
- **Anecdotal** reports have noted:
  —possible suppression of endogenous creatine synthesis (the making of creatine within the body)
  —possible enhanced renal stress/liver damage (short-term studies have shown no significant increase in blood tests that screen for kidney and liver damage)

—muscle cramps may result when exercising in the heat
—increased muscle strains and pulls may occur
—long-term effects are presently unknown

Currently, the scientific literature is lacking in this area, so anyone using creatine must do so with the understanding that long-term effects are not known. We will explore this in more detail later.

SUMMARY STUDIES

Juhn and Tarnopolsky, 1998: Mark Juhn, D.O., of the University of Washington, and Mark Tarnopolsky, M.D., of the University Medical Center in Hamilton, Ontario, Canada, published their papers "Oral creatine supplementation and athletic performance" and "Potential side effects of oral creatine supplementation: a critical review," in 1998 in the *Clinical Journal of Sport Medicine.* They found that "creatine supplementation is ergogenic in repeated 6–30-second bouts of maximal stationary cycling sprints." They also found that creatine improves strength for weight lifting.

In their study of side effects Juhn and Tarnopolsky found that the weight gain due to water retention from creatine supplementation "may impede performance in mass-dependent activities such as running and swimming." They added that short-term use of creatine supplements (twenty-eight days or less) does not appear to have adverse side effects, but they also noted that the studies involved very small numbers of test subjects. Consequently, they recommended large controlled studies for the future, so the effects of creatine supplements on the internal organs can be better evaluated.

THE BOTTOM LINE

Are you tired of reading about all these scientific studies? Do you just want the bottom line? What do all these studies add up to, anyway?

Here are a few conclusions:

• Creatine supplementation is ergogenic, meaning it can help to provide greater energy and lessen muscle fatigue.

• In the short term (up to eight weeks) creatine supplementation at recommended doses appears to have a positive effect on athletic performance when short bursts of intense activity are required.

• Creatine does not appear to have a beneficial effect on endurance sports, such as long-distance running and high jumping, possibly because it causes weight gain.

• Creatine supplements appear to work better when combined with glucose.

• Creatine supplementation does not increase energy or muscle mass for everyone.

• For short-term use creatine does not appear to have any dangerous side effects.

• Side effects such as cramping, diarrhea, and dizziness have been reported with creatine supplementation; studies are needed to find out if these side effects may be linked to dehydration or are the result of some other cause or causes.

• Studies are needed to find out if the increase in

muscle mass from creatine use is largely due to water retention or is, instead, mainly lean muscle growth.

• There is a great need for long-term studies involving large groups of test subjects. At this time long-term side effects of creatine supplementation remain unknown and current studies have employed very small numbers of participants.

• There is also a need for information on why individuals respond differently to creatine supplementation, whether rapid loading of creatine is more beneficial than gradual loading, and whether creatine use should be cycled.

Chapter 5

How Creatine Works

It's clear that we need energy in order to perform physical activities and that our muscles are a vital component in creating energy. We also know that the creatine stored in our muscles helps to fuel energy, and that stores can be increased by eating food with high creatine content, and especially by taking creatine supplements.

When creatine reserves are high many people find they have additional power and stamina to perform, especially when it comes to the short, intense bursts of energy required in so many sports.

In addition, supplementing with creatine over time appears to increase muscle size and diminish muscle fatigue, enabling us to be active longer and more effectively.

So you can conclude that if you use creatine regularly and also keep up your exercise or sports program on a regular basis, you have a better chance of improving your skills, increasing your muscle mass, and doing better in your fitness or sports program.

Does this mean you will turn into a champion overnight? Definitely not. But in some people and in some sports supplemental creatine can provide you with an edge.

But how exactly does creatine do its job? What goes on in the body, particularly in the muscles, that makes such a difference when there is extra creatine?

ENERGY SOURCES

In 1953 the Nobel Prize for Medicine and Physiology was awarded to two German-born scientists, Fritz Lipmann and Hans Krebs, for their individual studies of living cells. Krebs, a biochemist at Sheffield University in England, won the award for his work on energy. Specifically, he explained how sugar is converted into energy in the body through a chemical process now known as the Krebs cycle.

Krebs discovered that there is a series of complex chemical reactions involved in creating energy, and that these reactions all work toward creating adenosine triphosphate (ATP), the primary fuel for our muscle cells.

Basically, there are six components used by the body to create energy. They are ATP, creatine phosphate, glycogen, glucose, fatty acids, and amino acids. But of all these elements ATP is the one that actually provides the energy we all need to be physically active. As you will see, creatine is the most effective fuel to create ATP for specific types of exercise.

ATP AND ADP

When your body needs muscle strength to perform an activity, it breaks down ATP in order to convert it to adenosine diphosphate (ADP). This conversion releases energy. In the muscles the ADP then combines with the phosphocreatine (PC) stored there, and regenerates ATP, fueling strength in the muscles.

ATP is the fuel used by the body for the rapid, explosive type of energy needed in such sports as weight lifting, football, and baseball. Simply put, muscles are not able to contract without ATP.

Normally, muscles contain only enough ATP to provide energy for between five and ten seconds, depending on the amount of effort required for the activity. Then, the muscles need creatine to make more ATP.

The creatine in the muscles is of two main types:

- free creatine, which is chemically unbound, and represents about one third of the stores, and
- creatine phosphate, which represents about two thirds of the stores

It is creatine phosphate that is there to help when muscular ATP is quickly used up. The creatine phosphate breaks down and separates into creatine and phosphate, and the released energy regenerates ATP. The greater your stores of creatine, the more ATP your body can make to create energy for continuing your activities. But as you will see, there are limits to how much creatine your muscles can store, so you should definitely not conclude that more is better.

LENGTH OF EXERCISE

Note that we are saying that creatine is important for short-term high-intensity types of activity.

When the body needs fuel for a quick burst of energy, it uses the creatine stored in the muscles to make ATP. This burst of energy will use ATP and will last about five to ten seconds. So, for example, you could throw a discus or run fifty meters using the ATP present in your muscles at any given time.

Then, your body will take the stored creatine in your muscles and make more ATP for the next burst of energy, also lasting about five to ten seconds. This total energy output is enough to run a hundred-meter dash.

But after this ten to twenty seconds or so your phosphocreatine supplies drop markedly, and in an effort to create more ATP your body will begin to use its stores of glycogen and glucose. They will enable activity for about 120 seconds, but the energy they create is not as efficient as the creatine-generated energy, so your body may feel itself straining and beginning to get tired.

After this 120-second allotment of energy your body will gradually begin to go after fatty acids and amino acids as fuel. The energy they create is the type that permits long-term, aerobic endurance activities such as long-distance running. For these activities, unlike those that are short term and intense (and anaerobic), oxygen is needed.

As a general rule anaerobic activities tend to build big muscles, while aerobic activities do not.

WHEN CREATINE RUNS OUT

As we have seen, when muscles have used up their creatine supply and you still want to remain active, they must turn to other energy sources. Exactly how do they do this?

When creatine stores in the muscles are decreased and the body cannot regenerate enough in time, the body goes to its second choice: glycolysis. Glycolysis is the conversion of glucose (the end product of carbohydrate metabolism, which is stored in the liver and muscles as glycogen) to the simpler compounds lactate or pyruvate, in order to create ATP for energy.

Glycolysis also requires oxygen, which means you will have to breathe harder in an effort to get all the oxygen you need. The better condition you are in, the better you will be able to perform more work, but you still will not be able to get enough oxygen to perform the activities you want to do.

The problem is that when glycolysis takes place, there is a byproduct, lactic acid, which can cause pain and discomfort during intense activity and can also build up in the muscles and cause them to become fatigued or even to stop working altogether. Obviously, this situation, also known as "hitting the wall," can be very inconvenient if you're in the middle of an important game.

The bottom line is, creating energy using stores of creatine works much faster than the other options available to the body. When you need a quick burst of energy to start an activity or need several quick bursts to lift weights, make a basket, or score a hockey goal, creatine may be your best bet.

BENEFITS OF EXTRA CREATINE

Using creatine supplementation, you can obtain the following physiological benefits:

• More creatine phosphate will be available in the muscles to convert to ATP and create energy.
• Energy will be restored more quickly between bouts of activity, since ATP can rapidly regenerate.
• Muscles will not tire as quickly.
• Lower levels of lactic acid may be produced.
• Muscles will be able to grow (hypertrophy) due to increased activity.
• Extra fat may be lost due to increased activity.
• Benefits will be most obvious during and after short-duration, high-intensity activities.

So we see that by using supplemental creatine, we can increase the amount of creatine phosphate in the muscle cells and end up with more energy. If creatine works for you, you will soon see the difference in your performance, whether it's lifting weights in the gym, making a tackle, throwing a discus, or doing other similar, high-intensity actions.

But as we have already pointed out, the effects of creatine supplementation vary. Creatine simply doesn't work for everyone and it doesn't work in every sport or activity. Before you try it, it's a good idea to try to figure out if it might have any benefits for you.

Chapter 6

Sports Benefits of Creatine

By now you're probably saying, "All right. I understand that creatine helps create short bursts of energy. But is it going to help me in my sport or exercise routine?"

The answer is "Maybe. It all depends."

"On what?"

"On a lot of things. What sports you play, how you exercise, how often you're active, what you eat, your unique biochemistry, and probably some other unknown factors as well."

"Is it really all that complicated?"

"Yes and no. *After* you know all about creatine, if you think it might work for you, and you speak to a doctor, you can try it. That's the only way to know for sure."

AEROBIC AND ANAEROBIC EXERCISE

We've already mentioned these two basic types of exercise and defined them as:

Aerobic: exercise that requires the presence of
  oxygen; and
Anaerobic: exercise that does not require the
  presence of oxygen

We've also told you that the type of exercise where
creatine is especially important is anaerobic. But you
probably want to know a little more than that.

Aerobic exercise is long-term exercise that is usually
done in a repetitive, steady, low-intensity rhythm. It includes such activities as distance swimming, bicycle riding, in-line skating, walking, jogging, and long-distance
running. This type of exercise requires your heart and
your lungs to do a lot of work, and they can't do this
without oxygen.

As you do aerobic exercises, your circulatory system
sends oxygen to the large muscles you are using in your
arms, legs, back, and chest. That is why, when you have
exercised aerobically for a while, you may begin to
breathe heavily, especially if you are going beyond your
usual limits. Your body is trying to get more oxygen to
continue its work.

The main source of energy is the body's burning glucose and fat, which is only possible in the presence of
oxygen. Taking creatine with glucose may help improve
the levels of glycogen in the muscles. Glycogen is the
primary energy source for short-term aerobic activity.

Anaerobic exercise: Unlike aerobic exercise this form
of activity is usually short term, rapid, and high intensity. It includes weight lifting, sprinting, wrestling,

throwing (discus, javelin, shot put, hammer), and actions in many other sports, including football, basketball, baseball, and hockey.

Performing anaerobic exercise does not require the presence of oxygen. Rather, the short, intermittent, powerful bursts of energy that you need for anaerobic activity come from creatine helping to make ATP in your muscles.

But the division between these two is not so clearcut. They do overlap. For example, when you first begin an aerobic exercise, your body needs an extra boost and creatine is utilized. So strictly speaking, even though creatine is touted for its benefits on anaerobic activities, it also can theoretically help those doing aerobic activities, as well, but not nearly as much.

BUILDING MUSCLE

One of creatine's main effects on the body is to help build muscle. As you exercise normally, your muscles experience slight tears or damage, and in the presence of sufficient creatine, when the muscles repair themselves they also grow and develop in size.

More muscle means more strength and stamina.

That is why some of the greatest proponents of creatine supplementation have been bodybuilders. For people in this sport nothing is as important as building muscle, powerful, defined, buff muscle. And creatine really helps.

On the other hand, for people who need to run, swim, or cycle quickly over long distances, building muscle mass can be a disadvantage. Why? Because they also gain weight, and that can result in a slower pace and worsening performance.

WHAT CREATINE DOES FOR ATHLETES

Creatine has many positive effects that have made it the single most popular nutritional supplement for sports and fitness advocates. They include the following:

- increased muscle size
- greater physical strength
- longer endurance in short, repetitive activities
- less muscle fatigue
- increase in lean body mass
- shorter time for energy recovery
- greater muscle torque
- longer workouts and more reps

In their 1998 review study Juhn and Tarnopolsky summarized creatine's effects on various sports:

The data regarding creatine's ergogenic effects on mass-dependent activities, such as running and swimming, are not convincing, perhaps because of the side effect of weight gain from water retention. Studies on weight lifting suggest that creatine improves strength, possibly by increasing myofibrillar protein synthesis; however, more study is needed to prove this. No ergogenic effects on submaximal or endurance exercise are evident.

Individual response to creatine supplementation can vary greatly.

Unfortunately, most of the creatine studies to date have been laboratory studies and have not looked at actual athletes in the field. Until scientists have measured the effects of creatine supplementation on actual performance by amateurs and professionals involved in real competition or pursuing their exercise programs, it is difficult to gauge the exact value of added creatine.

The American College of Sports Medicine issued a position paper on creatine in 1998 and concluded that supplemental creatine helps athletes sustain their energy and strength during short-term maximal bouts of such activities as cycling, jumping, sprinting, and weight lifting.

The bottom line is this: if your exercise or sport benefits from added muscle mass, chances are creatine may work for you. But if additional weight or muscle is a problem, you're probably better off without it.

Now, let's look at specific sports and see how creatine may or may not be useful.

WEIGHT LIFTING

Lifting weights is the perfect activity for people supplementing with creatine. It requires a lot of strength and it occurs in brief, recurring rounds. In short, weight lifting is an anaerobic exercise that may improve with supplemental creatine.

People lift weights for many different reasons. They include the following:

- as part of an overall exercise program
- to build strength for a specific sport or activity
- to train as a competitive weight lifter or power lifter
- to maintain healthy bones
- to improve lean muscle mass
- to improve appearance
- to recover from an injury or illness
- to counteract the effects of aging

When you watch professional weight lifters, you see how they pause for a moment to collect themselves before attempting the lift. Both physically and mentally they are gathering all their power in order to be able to accomplish something that will take only a few seconds.

This is where creatine counts the most. Providing its help in the manufacture of ATP, creatine assists the muscles to attain maximum strength to lift very heavy weights in the prescribed manner.

Over time creatine supplements help weight lifters increase the size of their muscles and build up endurance, allowing them to work out for longer periods of time.

You may recall that the 1995 Earnest study used eight men who lifted weights and after using 20 grams a day of creatine monohydrate for twenty-eight days, the average man was able to lift an additional 8.2 kilograms, an improvement of 6.5 percent in less than a month. The number of reps they could do also increased significantly.

But creatine could also pose problems for weight lifters. In competitive weight lifting or power lifting there are different weight classes. Gaining weight, which can happen with the use of creatine, could make it difficult for someone to remain in that weight class. Therefore, if you are a competitor and do not want this to happen, the use of creatine supplements has to be carefully managed.

BODYBUILDING

The fact is, bodybuilders made creatine famous. Well before the media hype about Mark McGwire, every bodybuilder knew that taking creatine supplements was a big help in building and defining muscle.

Beyond a doubt creatine is the most popular supplement for bodybuilders. Why?

Because the ultimate goal of every bodybuilder is to make muscles grow to their maximum potential, so they are big and cleanly defined. In order to accomplish this bodybuilders need to reduce body fat and get muscles to grow. For these goals they use weight training, or resistance training.

As they lift progressively heavier and heavier weights, over a period of time their muscles incur minute damage and repair, each time growing in size and strength. That is, as long as all goes well and no injuries are sustained.

In order to avoid injury and exhaustion bodybuilders can train for only limited periods of time. But by adding creatine to their regimens bodybuilders are able to build muscle mass more quickly, which allows them to train longer and harder. The end result? Bigger, more defined, tougher muscles in less time.

FOOTBALL

First things first. Football players don't have to worry about their weight. Depending on the position played, added weight could even be an advantage. And of course, increased muscle mass and strength is a definite advantage.

In addition, football plays are fast, high intensity, and require sprinting, all of which is fostered by naturally produced creatine. Players will also benefit from increased stamina, allowing them to play longer and harder. And they will be able to recover more quickly from the abrupt bouts of explosive energy they need during the game.

Football players are also very prone to injury. It's a tough game. Creatine supplementation could theoretically make a difference in preventing injuries, due to less fatigue and enhanced muscle strength.

BASEBALL

Lots of baseball players are taking creatine, and some teams are even endorsing it or giving it to their players.

A lot of people think of baseball as a slow, leisurely game without the speed and intensity of other sports, such as football or basketball. But the main things in baseball are hitting, fielding, and pitching. All of these involve short-term rapid bursts of power, especially hitting.

Hitting a baseball also involves muscle power. Home-run hitters like Mark McGwire need the strength to hit a ball hundreds of feet time and time again. Here's where creatine may help to provide a boost.

Of course, not every baseball player will perform like McGwire. There are many more elements to his success than just the use of creatine and other supplements. For example, excellent eye-hand coordination is essential to good baseball performance, and creatine does not have any benefits for coordination. But it is feasible that the use of creatine could be a help to greater success.

But it's not only the power hitters who are using creatine. In 1997 Atlanta Braves pitcher Paul Byrd was quoted as saying, "You're seeing more pitchers using creatine. I think it's having a huge effect on baseball. I bet in five years every serious athlete will be taking it."

But the players taking creatine don't just swallow it and wait for miracles. They know that it's necessary to work out in order for the supplement to be effective. Today, professional baseball teams have trainers and conditioning programs that involve lifting weights and other strength-building activities. Many of these teams, like McGwire's St. Louis Cardinals, are making creatine available to their players on a regular basis.

To date no functional studies on creatine use in baseball have been done. So we can only extrapolate from lab studies to guess how creatine may help baseball players. There are many factors that affect baseball skills and it is difficult to determine whether or not creatine is beneficial. Although many baseball players seem to think it does help them, more research is definitely needed.

WRESTLING

Creatine supplements may be helpful for competitive wrestlers. Once again we have a sport that depends on quick, rapid, powerful movements. An ancient sport, wrestling's aim is to physically control your opponent.

It's true that physical strength and stamina are essential to success in wrestling, but it's not the whole story. The most powerful do not always win, because strategy, technical skills, psychological makeup, and many other factors are also important.

Then there are weight classes. Competitive wrestlers often diet in order to remain in their class, and weight gain is something they cannot afford.

Creatine can be a benefit in building muscular strength, endurance, and recovery. But it can be a major problem if it causes weight gain when it is not wanted.

Upper-weight or lighter-weight wrestlers who need to gain weight (which is uncommon) may benefit substantially from creatine. They can obtain benefits from gains in strength and weight.

But those who are dieting have to be careful during their competitive season. That is why many wrestlers may benefit by taking creatine during their off-season, when weight is not such an issue. These wrestlers should probably stop using creatine one month prior to the start of the season, so it can clear their system.

Wrestlers who want to consider using creatine in this way should, of course, consult a qualified health-care professional. And once again, more studies are needed in this area.

To sum up, wrestlers have to be careful about their

use of creatine. It's something each individual wrestler will have to work out under medical supervision.

TRACK AND FIELD

We've already seen in the studies discussed earlier that creatine is not helpful for long-distance sports or exercise, such as marathon running or distance swimming. But it can be very useful for short-term track-and-field events, such as running events up to eight hundred meters and throwing events with the discus, javelin, hammer, and shot put.

For example, in a 1997 study published in the *International Journal of Sports Medicine,* Bosco and his associates found that with creatine, jumping performance showed a 7-percent improvement during the first fifteen seconds of the jump test and a 5-percent improvement during the second fifteen seconds. Run time to exhaustion also increased by 13 percent.

In these short events competitors are called upon to demonstrate the kinds of short bursts of explosive energy that creatine helps to create.

In addition to their performance in competition, however, the positive effects of creatine can also help these athletes to train longer and harder, improving their skills.

SWIMMING

Although it is an aerobic activity, athletes involved in short-term competitive swimming, up to four hundred meters, appear to benefit from creatine supplements.

Here again the competitor is called upon to show

high levels of energy over a very brief period of time. Competitive swimmers also frequently take part in more than one event, and the extra creatine in their muscles can be an important factor in quicker recovery between events.

Studies on creatine supplementation in swimmers have added to our knowledge. For example, Grindstaff noted improved hundred-meter swimming time for those using creatine during the first two sprints, in his article "Effects of creatine supplementation on repetitive sprint performance and body composition in competitive swimmers."

However, Burke noted no changes in his study when there was a twenty-minute rest introduced, while Mujika noted a slight worsening with the use of creatine, which he thought might be due to weight gain.

Therefore, if you do short, rapid, repetitive swimming events, creatine might help, provided there isn't much rest in between your events. Otherwise you should be careful. You may instead want to try creatine during your off-season, when it is likely to provide help with your strength-conditioning program.

Remember that in swimming, as in some other sports, weight gain can be a deterrent, so swimmers who decide to use creatine will have to monitor their use carefully to make sure they do not gain any unwanted pounds.

CYCLING

Many studies have shown that with the use of creatine supplementation, there is improvement in cycling times for short sprints. However, just as many studies have shown a detriment for long-distance activity.

So once again, whether or not to use creatine will have to depend on what type of rider you are and what events you participate in. If you are just a recreational weekend rider, creatine use will probably not provide any noticeable benefits.

ROWING

Rowing is a sport that is becoming increasingly popular at the college and Olympic levels. Researcher Rossiter noted a two-second improvement in ergometer (indoor rower) scores in a thousand-meter rowing trial. This sport, like wrestling, has certain weight restrictions. Therefore, it may not be of value to use creatine *during* the rowing season.

If you are a rower and are interested in possibly using creatine, you should consult a qualified health-care professional for advice on its use, perhaps during the off-season.

KAYAKING

We have already seen how the 1998 study by L. R. McNaughton and associates showed that creatine supplementation significantly increased the amount of work done by test subjects using a kayak ergometer.

Again, it is best to consult your health-care professional to see if supplements of creatine, either in-season or off-season, can be of help if you partake in kayaking.

SOCCER AND BASKETBALL

Soccer is one of the most popular sports in the world. It is primarily aerobic and because of that, creatine supplements would not be of much help.

Basketball is very similar. However, certain positions, such as center, may require bigger mass and strength, so if you play center, creatine might be beneficial.

Again, a health-care professional should be consulted about possible use during off-season.

OTHER SPORTS

You can take what you know about how creatine works and apply it to your sport or exercise to try to determine if it would be helpful or not. At this point no one knows for certain, because no one has studied the use of creatine by actual athletes over any extended time period.

In order to try to decide you could ask yourself the following questions about your sport or exercise:

- Does it involve rapid bursts of energy?
- Is it mainly anaerobic or aerobic?
- Is added muscle mass an advantage or a disadvantage?
- Is additional body weight an advantage or disadvantage?
- Do I take part in my sport or work out on a regular basis (at least three times a week for at least thirty minutes)?

If creatine does not appear helpful for your sport, you might still benefit from its use during the off-season, in order to build up your strength or gain some of the other benefits we will be discussing.

Once you are familiar with the possible side effects and dangers of creatine supplementation, if you feel it might work for you and your medical professional agrees, you might want to try it and find out if it helps you. Whether you take karate classes once a week, play volleyball every summer at the beach, work out every weekend at the gym, or are in training to compete in archery at the Olympics, creatine can be an important part of your program.

The decision whether or not to use creatine is one that adults need to make, based on all the facts. Adolescents should definitely discuss this issue with their parents.

THE AMERICAN COLLEGE OF SPORTS MEDICINE

In 1998, after receiving many inquiries from their members and from the public, the American College of Sports Medicine (ACSM) decided to issue a position paper on creatine supplementation. The ACSM promotes and investigates scientific research, education, and practical applications of sports medicine and exercise medicine, and its members include doctors, trainers, and other sports professionals. The organization got together noted experts in the field in order to develop the position statement, which summarizes the information known about creatine and states their opinions about its use in sports.

Reviewing scientific literature, the ACSM concludes

that studies had "clearly shown that a regimen of creatine supplementation significantly enhances accumulation of creatine and phosphocreatine in skeletal muscle." The studies "indicate ingestion of 20–25 g creatine/day for 5–7 days decreases the normal decline in force or power production during short-duration, maximal bouts of exercise. Muscle creatine is maintained with a 3–5 g maintenance dose per day."

They point out that creatine supplements do not apparently improve performance of aerobic-type exercise, but that extra creatine may improve "recovery between bouts of exercise" and energy during "intense intermittent" activity.

A weight gain of between one and three pounds "is frequently observed after one week of creatine supplementation, attributable to an increase in total body water," they conclude. They also mention the fact that there is a lack of information on long-term use.

Who can benefit from using supplemental creatine? The ACSM paper says it is "those who participate in sports or activities that are short-term, intense bouts of exercise."

How does creatine supplementation change the stores in muscles? "A single 5-g dose of creatine consumed 4–5x/day (20–25g creatine/day) for 5–7 consecutive days enhances uptake of creatine into muscle by as much as 30%," the paper concludes.

What about people who skip the loading phase and go directly to the maintenance dose? "Lower dose supplementation with 3 g/day will also significantly elevate muscle creatine; however, the increase occurs gradually over several weeks rather than days," they state.

Dealing with the question of why some people seem to benefit from creatine while others do not, the ACSM states that "variability in creatine accumulation between individuals is quite large, which explains why some athletes may not experience an ergogenic effect. Individuals with lower total creatine values exhibit the greatest increases in creatine accumulation."

Discussing optimal doses, the paper says that once the levels of creatine in the muscle have been increased through supplements, "the breakdown occurs relatively slowly over about one month." For inactive people the ACSM recommends 2 grams per day, while those involved in resistance training should do well on a maintenance dose of 5 grams per day.

If this amount is good, would more be better? No, says the ACSM, stating that "there is no reason to believe that large doses would be necessary or beneficial to maintain elevated muscle creatine stores. Large doses of creatine consumed regularly may increase the incidence of potentially unknown detrimental side effects." In other words, remain cautious in your use of creatine, at least until more is known.

Specifically, what sports are enhanced by the use of creatine? The ACSM says that "creatine significantly enhances the ability to maintain power output during short-term maximal bouts of exercise, including cycling, sprinting, jumping, and weight-lifting protocols."

On the other hand, it has not been found especially

beneficial for "swimming, cycling, and longer-duration running protocols."

Noting reports of such side effects as "minor gastrointestinal distress, nausea, and muscle cramping," the paper observes that no negative side effects have been found in the scientific studies so far.

The ACSM position paper concludes that much additional research is needed in order to determine how to maximize creatine muscle stores, optimal doses, when and how to take creatine, why individuals vary in their responses, long-term effects, and how different groups respond, including women and the elderly.

Chapter 7

How to Buy Creatine

They call it "muscle candy," and health-food stores are having a hard time keeping it on their shelves. In fact, it's now showing up in supermarkets, convenience stores, drugstores, and every other place you can think of. Creatine is one of the most explosive products ever to hit the market and its popularity ratings, like the muscles it enhances, only seem to get bigger and bigger.

But if you want to try it, can you just hop into a store and buy some? How do you know which product to choose? There are hundreds of different ones, in every form imaginable.

Most of the creatine available is in powder form, ready to mix with liquids. But there are also tablets, capsules, gels, liquids, chewable wafers, candy bars, and chewing gum. Will lollipops be next?

It's all very perplexing. How do you know what to buy? Would one product be better for your needs than another? What about purity? Is it possible that different manufacturers (at different prices) are actually using the same creatine that they get from somewhere else? Where does this stuff come from, anyway, and how do they make it?

These are only some of the questions you should be asking before putting down your hard-earned dollars for a nutritional supplement that will be going into your body.

WHAT'S IN IT?

When creatine was first produced in the United States as a nutritional supplement in the late 1950s by the Illinois pharmaceutical company Pfanstiehl Laboratories, it was made by heating water and two chemical salts, cynamide and sarcosine.

Today, the supplemental creatine that you buy is organically synthesized from amino acids. As we know, the amino acids that naturally make up the creatine in our bodies are arginine, glycine, and methionine.

You should also know that pure creatine powder is odorless and tasteless, so if your product says it is pure creatine and it has an odor or a taste, you have reason to be suspicious.

Most of the manufacturers refuse to disclose exactly how they make creatine, considering it a trade secret. But a bigger secret is that many supplement companies do not make it at all. Instead, they buy it from mass producers, many of them in other countries.

The recent FDA regulation requiring detailed labeling on dietary supplements should help consumers to get more information on the contents of the products they buy. These labels must give listings for each separate ingredient and indicate how much of that ingredient is in each individual serving of the product.

But you, the buyer, will still not have all the information you need. You can try contacting the distributor's customer service department with some of these questions:

- Does the company manufacture its own creatine?
- If not, where does it get it?
- If so, what ingredients are used to make it?
- Why are other ingredients used and what are they for?
- Have tests been conducted for purity?
- Are there any ingredients included in the product that are not listed on the label?
- Does the product have any fillers?
- Will they send copies of tests and any other available information on their creatine product(s)?

Reputable supplement companies should be willing and able to answer your questions, but they may not be forthcoming about everything you want to know. And some companies will not respond at all.

So what should you do?

Your best and most practical bet is to purchase your creatine from a well-established, recognized supplement manufacturer that makes its own creatine and has the facilities and personnel to assure top quality.

If you're not sure which products fulfill these guidelines, ask your nutritionist, physician, or the owner of your local health-food store for advice.

This does not mean that the smaller or newer companies that sell creatine are giving you an inferior product. On the contrary, some of these products may even be superior to those of the older companies.

In addition, you can't totally believe every bit of the information you get from the companies that sell creatine, can you? Maybe they don't have the full information, maybe their information isn't correct and they don't even know it, maybe they don't want to tell you everything, or maybe they just want to hype their product.

So how can you know for sure?

There's really only one way: a lab test.

Of course, it may be difficult to find a lab that does a complete analysis of a nutritional product, but with persistence you should be able to find one. It is the only way you can know for certain what is in your creatine supplement.

But that's not the whole story. Any lab will tell you that every batch of a commercial product can be different. So just because you know what's in one batch, there's no guarantee the next batch you purchase will be identical.

Unfortunately, there is no perfect solution. But if you decide to use creatine, you should try to find a good, reputable product. Then, if it works for you and you get good results, stick with it.

FALSE LABELING

In 1998 Ray Sahelian, M.D., a creatine researcher and writer, drew attention to the results of a series of lab tests conducted by Alpha Chemical & Biochemical Laboratories, Inc., of California, an FDA-approved lab. A review of these tests was published by Advance Supplement Testing Systems in Mississippi.

The lab evaluated over 107 sports supplements, including a number of creatine products, and the findings indicate that 53 of these products, almost one half, deviated by 20 percent or more from the ingredient labels on their packaging.

As an example, Sahelian cites Muscle Tech's Creatine 6000-ES, Lot No. 972325, which claimed to contain 6 grams of creatine in each serving. The lab found that each serving actually contained only 2.25 grams of creatine, a very big discrepancy. They had similar findings for other supplements, including those containing protein, carbohydrate, and pyruvate.

Again, there is no way the consumer can make a judgment about possible false labeling unless the product is analyzed by an independent lab. And even then, it is possible that the lot analyzed was irregular in some way and that the rest of the distributor's products are properly labeled.

Finally, if you participate in organized sports and your creatine supplement has any banned substances, like andro, mixed in, it is possible that you could test positive in a random drug test and face very severe consequences.

THE COST

How much should you pay for your creatine?

That's not an easy question to answer, especially after

the information we've just seen about the possible differences in product quality.

While the most expensive product isn't always the best and the least expensive isn't always the worst, price does tell you something about quality.

So let's say you're not going to have lab tests done and you're going to stick with a creatine product made by a well-known company. About how much should you be paying?

There are quite a few factors to consider.

• *Are you buying in a store or through the mail?* Logic tells us that products purchased by mail should cost less because the seller has lower overhead. You can confirm this by comparison shopping. Go to a few stores and make a note of the price of the product you want to buy. Then check the mail-order prices. It may take a little time, but the savings over the long run can really add up.

• *Are you buying a product that is "pure" creatine or one that has other ingredients (which you may want)?* This can certainly affect the cost. It can either make it more expensive, if the added products cost more than creatine, or less expensive, if they don't. Remember that when you do this, you are getting less creatine for your money. Most people who buy these mixed products do so for convenience. They want to take several different substances for building muscle strength and energy, but don't want to be bothered taking them separately. So they let the supplement company combine them. If you really want to do your homework, you can check the prices of the separate ingredients (in the same dosages that you find in the mixed product) and see what you would be paying if you bought them individually. For some people the convenience of having them premixed is worth the extra cost. For others, it isn't.

• *Are you buying a product that the distributor makes in their own labs or one that they purchase from a mass producer?* If you are buying from a company that has its own labs and quality-control facilities, the chances are you will be paying a little more for your product. But this is not always so. Again, you need to check for yourself and then compare.

• *What form of creatine are you buying?* The form you buy can definitely affect the price. And it can also, more importantly, affect the amount of actual creatine you are getting. For example, a powder creatine product that contains only creatine monohydrate could be priced at seven cents a gram or two dollars per ounce. A liquid creatine, which also contains water, glycerine, flavoring, and citric acid, sells for about the same price. But the liquid, while more convenient since you don't have to mix it, is giving you much less creatine for your money.

On the other hand, creatine capsules, selling for about twenty-six and a half cents each, contain only 700 mg of creatine each, so you are paying a premium for the convenience of swallowing your creatine in capsule form. And you are getting barely three quarters of a gram of creatine. This compares to between five and a half cents and fifteen cents per gram charged for many mail-order creatine powders.

• *What size are you purchasing?* Supplement and food companies have become very erratic in the amounts in their packages, perhaps intentionally so. In the supermarket you can find tags that give you the price per ounce so you can compare different products. But you don't find those tags in the health-food store when you go to purchase creatine. So maybe you should bring a pocket calculator along with you to compare for yourself. The rule of thumb has always been that the bigger size is more cost effective, but that isn't always the case. Better to do the figures yourself and find out before you buy.

As an example, we calculated the price of three different sizes of the same creatine powder from one distributor. The smallest size, 210 grams, came out to about thirteen cents per gram, while the largest size, at 1,814 grams, came to five and a half cents a gram, quite a savings.

The bottom line: manufacturers of supplements do not have to prove their safety, purity, or effectiveness to any government agency before they can be sold. So people who purchase supplements really have to look out for themselves.

On average most people pay between thirty-five and fifty dollars per month, taking creatine at the recommended doses. When you buy, choose a product that says the contents are 99 percent creatine monohydrate and assures purity.

By now you may be thoroughly confused and maybe even disgusted. So if you decide you want to try creatine, why not ask your friends, your physician, nutritionist, trainer, or health-store manager to make some recommendations? Lots of people have been using creatine for years and many of them swear by one specific product that they say has worked well for them. So instead of making a time-consuming scientific study, you might simply decide to collect some firsthand information from real people and go from there.

And while it's true that people are buying $200 million worth of creatine a year, many of these people may not know what they're doing. They may be getting inferior products or using something they don't really need or that isn't effective or that could cause problems for them. Or maybe they aren't using their creatine in the most effective way. So it might be a good idea to step back from the creatine craze and exercise a little caution before you jump in.

Chapter 8

How to Use Creatine

So you decide you want to use creatine. You go out, buy some, and follow the instructions on the package. Right?

Maybe.

Because even though creatine is the most widely used, and apparently one of the safest, of the muscle-enhancing supplements, it's still somewhat controversial.

For example, not everyone agrees that it's a good idea to take it. And not everyone agrees on the best way to take it.

There are questions about optimal doses, about whether or not to load, and about whether or not to cycle.

Experts have different opinions regarding when to take it, what to mix it with, and whether to use pure creatine or products with other ingredients.

There's also some debate about whether certain foods or beverages help or hinder creatine's effectiveness.

Experts also have different explanations about why creatine doesn't seem to work at all for certain individuals.

And then there are some people who shouldn't use creatine at all. You might be one of them.

All of these factors are important considerations for determining whether or not to use this dietary supplement and, if you do, exactly how you use it.

GETTING PROFESSIONAL ADVICE

Before you make your decision about whether or not to use supplemental creatine, or before you determine whether or not you should continue to use it if you're already taking it, it's important to get some professional advice.

The first person you should ask is your physician. Chances are, with all the publicity surrounding creatine, your doctor knows something about it and can advise you on whether or not it's a good idea for you to use it.

If your doctor is not familiar with creatine, you could ask him or her to do some research or to refer you to a physician who is familiar with sports supplements. Most often, a primary-care sports medicine specialist will be the best person to consult for advice.

Next, if you use the services of a registered dietician/nutritionist or a certified athletic trainer, consider getting his or her advice. Some of the questions you might want to ask are:

• Do you think I should be using creatine supplements?

- How much should I take each day?
- Should I load up when I first start?
- Should I cycle?
- When should I take my supplements?
- What should I take creatine with?
- Could creatine react badly with any other supplements or medications I'm taking (including over-the-counter drugs)?
- Do I have any health problems that might mean I shouldn't be using creatine?
- What's the maximum amount I should take and for how long?
- Can you recommend any specific brands?
- Have you ever used creatine and if so, what has it done for you?

We will go over all these issues to help you make your own decision. But it is still very important for you to get the advice and have the monitoring of your medical professional. You can add to your knowledge by getting additional information from others, including nonmedical professionals and your friends, but don't rely completely on their advice—it could be wrong, incomplete, or just not right for you.

HOW MUCH TO TAKE

The amount of creatine you take will depend on several factors, including your decision on whether or not to load when you first begin using it, which we will discuss shortly.

Apart from your possible initial loading period the

average recommended dose of creatine is 5 grams a day, which gives you the equivalent of the creatine in about two and a half pounds of lean beef. Five grams is what you usually get in one teaspoon of powdered creatine.

However, many people who are active in sports take higher amounts, more in the general range of 20 to 25 grams per day. At least for a period of time.

Creatine researcher Anthony Almada of the University of Nebraska suggests that people involved in regular high-intensity activities take 10 to 15 grams of creatine daily, no matter how much they weigh. He says that further studies should provide more exact information.

On the lower end of the scale Pfanstiehl Laboratories, one of the largest producers of creatine in this country, recommends a dosage of between 2 and 5 grams a day.

One of the factors affecting your determination on how much to take is your body weight.

If you want to use this method of calculating your daily intake, the following chart can help you to determine the optimum creatine dose for your body weight.

SUGGESTED DAILY AMOUNT OF SUPPLEMENTAL CREATINE

Body Weight	Percent of Body Fat				
	4%	8%	12%	16%	20%
	Grams Per Daily Serving of Creatine				
114	5	4.75	4.5	4.25	4
123	5.5	5	5	4.75	4.5
132	5.75	5.25	5	5	4.75
148	6.5	6.25	6	5.75	5.5
165	7.25	7	6.75	6.5	6.25
181	7.75	7.5	7.25	7	6.75
198	8.5	8.25	8	7.75	7.5
220	9	8.75	8.5	8.25	8
242	10.5	10.25	10	9.75	9.5
275	11	10.75	10.5	10.25	10
300	12	11.75	11.5	11.25	11

Adapted from chart provided by Twin Laboratories, Inc.

So to help you determine exactly how much creatine you need, you can consider the following factors:

- your body weight (heavier people often use more)

- your percentage of body fat (lean people use more)
- your level of physical activity
- the intensity of your activities
- how big your muscles are (bigger muscles can store greater amounts of creatine)

You should also be aware that the total amount of creatine in the recommended dose of each company's product can be different, and within one company each separate creatine product may also have different amounts of creatine in each teaspoonful.

Most powders of pure creatine are standardized to provide 5 grams per teaspoon, but it is still a good idea to check the label to make sure that's what you're getting.

Different forms of the product, other than powder, also vary. For instance, one liquid product has 2,500 mg (2.5 grams) in each teaspoon, while another liquid has only 1.5 grams. So you have to be careful to read the label to see how much creatine you are getting in each teaspoon and adjust the number of teaspoons you take accordingly, in order to get the amount you want.

Dosages also vary with capsules. One creatine producer sells capsules with 750 mg of creatine, while another has 700 mg, both less than one gram.

And when it comes to wafers and candy bars, of course, the amount of actual creatine you get will be far less.

The exact amount you use can also depend on how

much intense activity you perform. Within the recommended dosage of between 2 and 20 grams of creatine a day, you should be able to find your ideal daily intake.

The bottom line? Read the label, know what you're getting, follow your doctor's advice, and monitor your progress carefully. And remember that no one knows exactly what the optimum dosage of creatine is for each person; it varies from person to person, and it will probably take several years of scientific studies to come up with better guidelines for the public.

But you should keep in mind that when it comes to taking creatine, more is not better. Once your muscles are saturated with creatine, they can't take in any more. Additional supplies will be converted to creatinine and excreted in your urine. You also run the risk of experiencing unwanted side effects. So be cautious and do not overdo your intake. It is far better to take too little creatine than to take too much.

LOADING

A review of the literature indicates that many experts think loading is a good idea. At least for most people. However, it may not be right for everyone and there are many experts who say it isn't even necessary to begin with. Opinion is very divided.

Loading means taking a larger amount of a substance when you first begin in order to load up or saturate your tissues with it, bringing them up to maximum levels. Then, after a few days of taking higher doses, you go into a maintenance phase, where you begin to take a lower daily amount.

Some people say that loading creatine isn't necessary and only winds up costing you more money. They claim that the extra creatine you take for the first few days will only be excreted, giving you no benefit, and it could also put a strain on your organs, which are not used to processing such large amounts.

But proponents of loading say it's a good idea because if you're physically active and doing the kinds of exercise or sports that involve short bursts of intense energy, your creatine stores are probably too low and need building up. Loading creatine will give you an immediate boost, getting your energy up, and then when you go on the maintenance dose, you will be in better condition to continue with the same level of intense activity.

Some experts advocate loading because they believe muscle uptake of creatine is at its greatest when you first start taking the supplement, and that maximal amounts of the substance can be stored during this period.

The other factor to consider is individual differences among people. We already know that vegetarians have lower levels of creatine in their bodies to begin with, so loading might be good for them. But creatine doesn't work for everyone and for those it does help, effects may vary. So we still need to do a lot more research to come up with clearer answers.

You can get similar effects by skipping the loading phase and instead taking a lower dose over time. However, it does take longer. In 1996 Dr. Eric Hultman and his colleagues in Nottingham, England, published their findings of a study on this topic in *The Journal of Applied Physiology*.

Entitled "Muscle creatine loading in men," the report concluded that after twenty-eight days, one group of test subjects who had loaded 20 daily grams of creatine for the first six days and then gone on the maintenance dose of 3 grams per day had the same levels in their bodies as another group who had not loaded and had taken 3 grams a day throughout.

So while loading may possibly give you an initial burst of energy, it probably does not increase your creatine stores over a period of weeks.

But if you decide that you want to load when you begin using creatine, here's what to do:

• Take 20 to 30 grams of creatine each day (depending on your weight and other needs).
• Divide your total creatine intake into four to six separate servings of no more than 5 grams at a time.
• Take your four to six doses throughout the day (see p. 88 for suggestions on when to take them).
• Do this for five to seven days.
• Then lower your daily creatine intake to between 2 and 5 grams per day (or more, depending on your weight and other needs).

Dr. Richard Kreider has recommended maintenance doses of 0.03 grams per kilogram of body weight, to be adjusted as needed. Using this formula, a person weighing 150 pounds (68.04 kilograms) would take about 2 grams of creatine a day, while someone weighing 200 pounds (90.72 kilograms) would take 2.75 grams. This recommendation is lower than the commonly used 5 grams per day. (One pound is equal to .4536 kilograms and one kilogram is equal to 2.2046 pounds, in case you want to calculate your own weight.)

Loading does have one theoretical side effect. By flooding your body with high levels of creatine, you may be stressing your kidneys and your liver too much. In addition, once muscles are saturated, additional creatine is excreted as the waste product creatinine. So there are some who think loading is not only unnecessary, but potentially harmful to the body. Therefore, since scientists do not have all the information on the side effects of creatine, it may be best to use the lower doses and avoid the loading phase entirely.

If you decide that you do not want to load, that you don't need a sudden, extra burst of power and can be patient and wait for results over a period of weeks, you can just begin taking from 2 to 5 grams of creatine per day, based on your weight, and maintain this steady intake. But you should be careful not to skip any doses, because if you do, you will lose the effectiveness of this method.

It takes from fourteen to twenty-eight days of not taking creatine for your body to return to its normal creatine levels. That is one reason why you do not want to skip any doses. If you do stop taking creatine for more than two weeks and you are using the loading method, you should consider reloading to bring your creatine levels back up.

WHEN TO TAKE CREATINE

What's the best time to take your creatine doses? Before, after, or between meals? When you first get up, before going to bed, or some other time? And how long before and after exercising?

Many experts advise taking creatine before and after workouts for these reasons:

• Creatine right before exercise appears to more effectively saturate the muscles, maximizing stores and providing energy for your activities.

• Creatine right after exercise will replenish the depleted stores of creatine that you have used for your exercise or sport.

So if you are dividing your doses into four or five per day during the loading phase, make sure that at least two of them are used before and after your workout.

Although some companies advise taking creatine between meals, others say it's all right to take it with meals or that it doesn't matter. Since we get our natural stores of creatine from the meat and fish and animal products we eat, there's really no reason why creatine supplements should not be taken along with food.

In addition, as we will see, some people experience side effects when they take creatine, including intestinal gas, cramps, and diarrhea. For some of these people, taking creatine with meals appears to ease such reactions.

Until studies have come up with a definitive answer, you should experiment and see whether you get better effects by taking your creatine supplements with your meals or separately.

WHAT TO MIX WITH CREATINE

If you buy your creatine in powder form, as most people do, you will have to mix it with three or four ounces of liquid.

Creatine powder can be mixed most easily with water or juice. Most experts recommend using juice, particularly grape juice, because of its high carbohydrate content, including natural sugars.

The reason? Absorption of creatine is faster when it is taken with glucose (a sugar), because it raises the levels of insulin in your body. In fact, some creatine producers are now adding glucose to their creatine products.

Many fruit juices are good to mix with creatine, but grape juice, which is high in dextrose (a form of glucose, also called "grape sugar"), is the liquid favored by many creatine experts. The reason is that combining creatine with a high-carbohydrate liquid like grape juice speeds its entry into the bloodstream, raising blood glucose and insulin levels, and allowing the creatine to reach your muscles more quickly.

Of course, you can also use grape juice to swallow your creatine tablets or capsules, if that's the form you've chosen.

In regard to the liquid and gel forms, there has been some controversy over whether or not they break down once the bottle is opened. For that reason this form of creatine has not sold very well. But if you decide to try them, the producers' instructions are to take them alone, not mixed with any other liquids. Most gels have carbohydrates already mixed in and the liquid is supposed to be taken sublingually (under the tongue) so it will be more quickly absorbed.

You may also want to consider taking creatine with a glycogen replacement drink or an electrolyte replacement drink. This can be of help in other areas of your sports performance, especially endurance.

INTERACTIONS

How does creatine mix with other substances, including the food you may eat with it? Are there any things you should stay away from? Again, to be completely safe, it is always best to consult your personal physician.

Supplements: If you are taking other supplements, including vitamins, minerals, and herbs, there is no evidence that taking creatine will have any adverse effects, provided they are taken at recommended levels.

Prescription drugs: So far, studies have not found any adverse reactions in people taking prescription medication as directed, and creatine. Check with your doctor to be sure.

Caffeine: Combining creatine with caffeine could be a problem. In 1996 K. Vandenberghe and his colleagues published a paper entitled "Caffeine counteracts the ergogenic action of muscle creatine loading" in *The Journal of Applied Physiology.* The paper reported on their study of the effects of caffeine on creatine supplementation.

The researchers found that their test subjects, divided into three groups, performed physical activities best when taking only creatine. The group that took creatine plus 400 mg of caffeine performed less well, and was about at the same level as those who took a placebo (and no creatine or caffeine).

Although this is only one study and used a very small number of men, it is indicative that the full ergogenic benefit of creatine supplementation can be obtained by those who do not use caffeine-containing beverages or food, especially if caffeine intake is high. The 400 mg dose of caffeine is the equivalent of about six cups of instant coffee or three and a half of brewed.

Does it mean that if you're using creatine, you have to give up caffeine completely? Probably not, but it would be a good idea to keep your consumption of caffeine-containing items in the moderate range. These include not only coffee and tea, but many soft drinks, as well as chocolate.

There are also studies that show that moderate amounts of caffeine have benefits in terms of mental alertness and energy. So which is better: moderate caffeine or none at all? Your best bet is to find out, through experimentation, what works for you.

CYCLING

Should you take creatine steadily, at your established daily dose (regular or maintenance) for the foreseeable future, or is it better (and wiser) to stop taking it at certain intervals? *Cycling* is the term to describe the procedure of taking something for a while, then stopping and going off it for a specific period of time, then taking it again. Whether or not you should cycle creatine is another decision you will need to make.

Cycling was really popularized by athletes taking dangerous steroids. Knowing that steroids were not beneficial for their bodies, people taking them thought they could get a measure of protection by letting their bodies have a break from steroids and get back to normal before they hit them with another round of these drugs. In addition, as we will see, steroid use can result in very unpleasant side effects and the athletes using steroids were trying to lessen them.

But creatine, to the best of our knowledge, is not dangerous when taken as recommended. If you saturate your muscles with creatine during regular use and then stop, but still continue with your rigorous activities, your muscle stores will return to normal and your energy and strength may drop back, depending on how long you go without creatine supplements.

Then, in order to get back where you were when you stopped taking it, you will have to go through a loading period again. Does that make sense?

It could.

Remember that your body makes 1 to 2 grams of creatine daily and you do not want to shut that mechanism off permanently. There are some researchers who think that using supplemental creatine could interfere with the body's natural ability to make creatine and that cycling gives the body a chance to function naturally again.

So far there are no studies that show this happening,

but it is a good idea to be cautious until studies confirm whether or not this occurs. They also point out that there are no long-term studies on the effects of creatine and there is always the possibility that regular use could have some harmful effects.

If you do decide to cycle, experienced creatine users recommend different forms of cycling, including these patterns:

• Take creatine for eight weeks; stop taking creatine for four weeks; then resume creatine for another eight weeks, and so on.
• Take creatine every other day.
• Take creatine seven days, then stop taking it for the next seven days.
• Take creatine for three months, then go off it for one month.
• Load for five to seven days, go on maintenance for thirty to forty days, stop for three to five weeks, then begin again.

If you want to cycle, does it matter which one you choose? Probably. The most important factor is for you to work around your training schedule. At the times that you want to build up your strength, or when you are doing a lot of anaerobic activity, you should stay on a good dose of creatine with or without a loading phase.

For example, if you participate in an aerobic sport, you could stay on creatine for a few months when you might be emphasizing your weight training, then go off it for one month prior to your competitive season. It is important for you to look at your total training program over a full year, with the help of a health-care professional, in order to figure out how to best use creatine.

It is also probably best to remain on the cautious side. That means taking a break for a month or two at a time every three months or so. Again, this has to be timed with your individual sports season (preseason, in-season, postseason, and off-season) so you have a plan that is effective for you.

Finally, we should add that there are anecdotal reports from some athletes using creatine who cycle indicating that if they go off creatine for a few weeks before a major competition, then go through the loading period and onto their maintenance dose, they appear to get a renewed burst of energy in their activities beyond what they had when they were not cycling and were taking a regular, steady dose.

WHY CREATINE MAY NOT WORK

So far, creatine sounds like a miracle for anyone who wants to build muscle, increase strength and energy, and do it in a quick, safe way.

But remember that way back at the beginning of this book, we mentioned that creatine works for approximately 80 percent of the people in studies showing benefits. What about that other 20 percent? Why didn't creatine work for them?

Again, no one has definitive answers. More and longer studies are needed to find the reasons why. But that hasn't stopped creatine researchers and others from speculating.

Here are some of the possible reasons why creatine might have no effect on certain people:

• They have naturally high stores of creatine in their muscles already (possibly from their diets), and taking supplements does not appreciably increase these reserves. Remember that there is a limit to how much creatine your muscles can hold and when that limit is reached, any excess is excreted from the body.

• They are largely sedentary and do not exercise much. Remember that usually, the positive effects of creatine are only felt when supplementation is accompanied by physical activity.

• They engage in aerobic exercise and do not partake in sports or activities that require the short bursts of high-intensity action that are benefited by extra stores of creatine. Remember that performance in long-distance low- or moderate-intensity exercises such as marathon running may actually suffer with creatine use because the increased muscle mass and weight may slow down the athlete.

• They have some biochemical characteristic that prevents their bodies from processing supplemental creatine to create greater muscle mass and energy.

• They may not have taken enough creatine in the studies and may need to have their dose reevaluated.

• They may need to take the creatine with some additional substance, such as glucose, for maximum effectiveness.

So if you're among the 20 percent who try creatine and find it doesn't work for you, chances are, it's probably not something you should worry about.

But before you draw any conclusions, you should first review your dose, exercise regimens, and the other aspects of your training program. Make sure that your expectations are in line with what the studies tell you to expect in terms of performance enhancement from creatine use. Then, when you are certain that everything else is right and you are still not benefiting, you may simply be a "nonresponder."

If so, you can continue with your regular workouts, most likely with power and stamina similar to those who are "responders." Remember, you cannot lose the hard work that you did while exercising.

WHO SHOULD NOT USE CREATINE

If you don't respond to creatine supplementation after trying it for a while, if you experience unwanted side effects, or if there are other reasons you do not like the supplement, you are unlikely to become a regular user.

But are there any people who should not even try it? Who might find it dangerous to their health? Yes, there are.

Again, we remind you to consult your physician or other qualified health-care professional before you begin taking supplemental creatine. Make sure your doctor is familiar with any health problems you may have, your personal and family medical history, and any medications you may be using.

• People with kidney problems should probably not use creatine.

• People with liver problems should probably not use creatine.

• People taking drugs that affect the liver or kidney should be very careful about their use of creatine and should only use it under medical supervision.

• Young children should probably not use creatine.

• Teenagers should probably only use small amounts and for a limited period of time (such as a few months) and only after consultation with a doctor and their parents.

• Pregnant women or women wanting to become pregnant should avoid taking creatine.

In addition, as you will see shortly, creatine can have many potential side effects and that can also affect your decision about whether or not you should be using it.

If you and your doctor decide that you should try creatine, even though there are health concerns, be certain that you are carefully and regularly monitored for any possible negative reactions.

Chapter 9

Creatine for Your Health

As we've pointed out, creatine is one of the most studied nondrug substances in history. Its effectiveness in building muscles and providing vigor and strength to athletes, and its apparent lack of serious side effects, have excited scientists who are eager to know more about it.

So in addition to the approximately two hundred scientific studies that have been done so far, many others are ongoing or planned for the near future. And one of the most interesting aspects to all this research is the fact that it's uncovered additional benefits for creatine, many of them directly related to our physical health.

PHYSICAL CONDITIONING

While the direct result of creatine supplementation is to build muscle size, strength, and stamina, there are also some significant indirect results.

• Because skeletal muscle is attached to bone, people who use creatine and *exercise* may find that over time they have *stronger bones* and experience *fewer fractures.*

• Creatine helps build lean muscle and may help with the *loss of excess body fat* around the muscles.

• Because creatine improves performance, athletes tend to exercise more and for longer periods of time, giving them the benefits of *frequent and full workouts.*

• Added strength and stamina can also improve *sexual performance,* leading to a more satisfying physical relationship with one's partner.

ILLNESSES AND DISEASES

Researchers have also found benefits using creatine supplements for certain health conditions.

• *Lou Gehrig's disease:* Two studies published in early 1999 both found that creatine supplements helped to build up muscles in people with Lou Gehrig's disease, also known as amyotrophic lateral sclerosis (ALS), a fatal condition that results in progressive degeneration of motor neurons and muscular strength.

The first study, reported in the journal *Neurology,* concluded that 5 to 10 grams of creatine per day resulted in a 10- to 15-percent improvement in the muscular strength of patients with various neuromuscular disorders.

The second study, published in *Nature Medicine,* found that supplemental creatine given to mice with Lou Gehrig's disease improved their physical endurance and also extended their lives. In fact, one

study found that creatine was twice as effective as rilu-
zole, the only FDA-approved medication used to treat
this disease, which can cost up to $12,000 per year.

The researchers, from Harvard Medical School and
Cornell University Medical College in Manhattan,
were funded by the National Institutes of Health, the
Muscular Dystrophy Association, and the ALS Association.

Of course, just because this one study had good results in mice, it does not necessarily mean that creatine supplements will have the same effects on human
patients. But it is a hopeful sign for the approximately
thirty thousand Americans who have ALS.

Since most people with ALS live for only about
four years following their diagnosis, it is likely that
many of them will try creatine supplementation, while
waiting for the outcome of further studies.

• *Other neuromuscular diseases:* Because of creatine's positive effect on muscular strength, it is also
quite possible that it could be useful in treating other
neuromuscular diseases, such as Parkinson's disease,
muscular dystrophy, multiple sclerosis, and Hunting-
ton's disease, as well as AIDS.

In fact, led by Mark Tarnopolsky, M.D., Canadian
researchers at McMaster University Medical Center in
Hamilton, Ontario, tested creatine supplements on
patients with muscular dystrophy and other neuromuscular diseases. According to their results, published in the journal *Neurology* in 1999, between 10
and 20 percent of the patients showed improvement

on tests to measure their muscular strength, and this improvement was on average 15 percent.

The group included eighty-one patients who had low levels of creatine in their muscles, which was determined by a muscle biopsy. The researchers gave the test subjects 5 grams of creatine twice a day for ten days, and then tested them to find out if there was any improvement in the strength of their hand grasp and their ability to lift their knees and to pull up their feet.

For most patients with muscular dystrophy and similar neuromuscular diseases, there is a loss of about 10 percent in muscle strength per year. Therefore, an improvement of 15 percent in a short period of time with the use of supplemental creatine is quite significant. The researchers have been working with this group for about a year and intend to continue following them.

• *People who cannot make creatine:* There are some people who have disorders that prevent them from making creatine in their bodies properly, and as a result their stores are very low. These people appear to do much better when they are given supplemental creatine.

• *Muscular weakness in the elderly:* In the same way, creatine could be of great benefit to older people whose muscles have begun to weaken through the natural process of aging. By combining creatine supplements with a regular exercise program, muscles could not only be strengthened, but the large number of fractures resulting from falls in the elderly could theoretically be lowered.

CHOLESTEROL LEVELS

There are two types of cholesterol in the body: the "good kind" or HDL (high-density lipoproteins) and the "bad kind" or LDL (low-density lipoproteins). So what you want to do, of course, is keep the bad cholesterol levels down and the good ones up.

Cholesterol is a waxy substance that builds up in your arteries, accumulating in the walls of blood vessels and in your heart and impeding blood flow, which can lead to heart attacks and strokes. But as we explained, there are actually two components of cholesterol: LDL, the bad type that clogs the arteries, and HDL, the good type that helps carry the LDL out of the body.

Experts say that at least 25 percent of your total cholesterol should be HDL. In general, people who are physically active and exercise a lot tend to have higher HDL levels than people who do not. But there are also other contributing factors, such as diet, heredity, and stress.

At one point in the past people were being told that total cholesterol levels over two hundred were dangerous and had to be reduced through low-fat, low-cholesterol diets, and/or medication. Today, there is not as much agreement about this and there is often more emphasis on the ratio of HDL to LDL than on the total reading.

Creatine has been reported to benefit cholesterol profiles (total cholesterol and HDL/LDL ratios) in middle-aged men and in trained men and women with high levels of triglycerides (fat particles). C. P. Earnest's 1996 study showed that creatine decreased levels of total cholesterol by 6 percent and triglycerides by 22 percent. Kreider also noted increases of 13 percent in HDL with the use of creatine.

Because of its apparent beneficial effects on cholesterol levels, creatine may provide additional cardiovascular benefits. More research will have to be done before we can determine exactly why this may occur, and to confirm results.

Can you use creatine to lower your own cholesterol levels?

Again, this is something to discuss with your doctor. But if you decide that you are going to supplement with creatine, it might be interesting and beneficial to have your cholesterol levels measured before you begin and then again a few months later, so you can compare the results.

Recovery from Surgery

We have seen how creatine benefits physically active people by maximizing creatine stores in the muscles. We have also seen that it does not do much for people who are sedentary.

But what about people who have been forced to give up all their physical activities for a while and then have to try to regain their lost strength?

Surgical patients who have been in bed for some time usually have some degree of difficulty getting their mobility back. Being forced to stay off your feet or only move slowly with assistance while you are recovering can be very bad for maintaining normal muscular vigor. In addition, such patients often lose a lot of weight, and creatine can help to prevent this loss.

And few things are worse for the dedicated fitness enthusiast than losing physical dexterity and power.

Here's where creatine can be a real help.

By using creatine supplements while you are recovering from surgery, you can give your muscles a much-needed boost to get them back in shape. By providing extra stores of fuel for energy, you will accelerate the healing process and shorten your recovery period.

Heart Disease

One area of creatine research that is not discussed too often but is highly researched is its use intravenously in patients with severe heart disease. This intravenous use of phosphocreatine can decrease ventricular fibrillation (a deadly heart rhythm) and can also help to improve the heart's metabolism. Because of this researchers are now studying the effects of oral creatine on heart function to find out if any similar benefits may result.

And as studies continue, it is likely that researchers will uncover additional physical benefits of supplemental creatine.

Chapter 10

Side Effects and Dangers

We keep calling creatine one of the best and apparently safest supplements around. But that doesn't mean that it's completely safe, that it's safe for everyone, or that we know everything about it.

There are many concerns about using creatine, and it's important for you to be informed about its possible side effects and dangers before you decide to use it.

NO LONG-TERM STUDIES

We have already mentioned that the lack of long-term studies is a major concern that many people have about using creatine. How do we know for sure that it is safe?

The answer is, we don't.

Remember that creatine is a supplement, not a drug, and is not regulated by the FDA. As a consequence the rigorous testing that drug companies have to go through in order to prove the safety and effectiveness of their products, and that often costs many millions of dollars, has not been done with creatine.

But, as we have seen, many studies have been carried out by very reputable scientists over a period of years. Unfortunately, these studies rarely exceed time periods of more than eight weeks.

Eight weeks of studying the effects of creatine supplements on the human body are simply not sufficient for us to draw conclusions about its effects over time.

Many substances can appear safe when used for a few weeks or months or even for a few years. But it's also possible that after ten years of steady use, some health problems can develop.

Just look at tobacco use, for example. It's very hard to get teenagers to stop smoking, because the serious health effects of smoking can take twenty or more years to appear.

To date our longest rigorous scientific studies are two years or less in length. So until we have studies on people using creatine for periods of five, ten, fifteen, or twenty years, we cannot say for certain that using it is entirely safe.

DEHYDRATION

One of the things creatine does is to draw water into the muscles. That's one reason why with time, muscles become larger and harder. And that's why it's so important to take your creatine supplements with plenty of liquids and to keep up the intake of liquids throughout the day to replenish the water that is drawn into the muscles and the water that is lost during exercise.

Dehydration can become a really serious problem when people take more than the recommended doses.

Houston Astros outfielder Derek Bell was hospitalized twice in 1998 for kidney problems that he reportedly says are related to his heavy use of creatine.

And it has been reported that Brady Anderson of the Baltimore Orioles says that he, too, uses much higher than recommended doses, but he also says that he drinks at least a gallon of water a day.

To avoid dehydration and the possibility of damage to your kidneys or other organs, be certain to take your creatine only in recommended doses, accompanied by plenty of water and other fluids.

If you do get dehydrated a lot or if you practice excessively in hot, humid environments, you should consider not using creatine at all. For example, in football camps, where there is athletic practice twice a day in heavy equipment and hot weather, creatine can be a problem. The more dehydrated you become, the harder your kidneys have to work and the greater your potential for creatine to have bad effects on your kidneys.

POSSIBLE SIDE EFFECTS

Many people experience no side effects when using creatine, but others complain of a variety of symptoms that they find unpleasant, uncomfortable, or unacceptable.

These include the following:

- dehydration
- diarrhea
- cramps
- intestinal gas

- headaches
- nausea
- dizziness
- muscle pulls or sprains
- stress on the kidneys and/or liver
- weight gain

Some of these side effects can be a result of taking creatine in higher amounts than the body can easily process. Remember that every person is different and just because your friends can take 10 grams a day without problems, it doesn't mean that you can do the same.

So the first thing to do when you experience these side effects is to consult your doctor and then either:

- stop using creatine for a while
- try it at a lower dosage
- increase your liquid intake
- take your creatine with your meals or vary dose times, or
- take smaller amounts in more doses throughout the day

When it comes to muscle pulls or sprains, there is really no current scientific evidence to suggest that creatine causes these problems. A more likely explanation is that the increased strength people attain with creatine use leads them to exercise more, perhaps to the point of exhaustion, where injuries are far more common. Or it may give them the idea that they can do more than they really can, leading them to put too much pressure on their muscles.

Some even think that the muscles may get big too fast with the use of creatine. As the tendons and ligaments try to adapt, increased strain can result. While preliminary studies have not shown an increase in muscle injuries, more research needs to be done.

There are some experts who feel that the other side effects listed are also not directly connected to creatine use, but are instead results of dehydration and exhaustion due to exercise, especially under hot and humid conditions.

In addition, we have already mentioned the most common side effect, which is *weight gain.* It can be a problem for people in certain sports, such as long-distance running, high jumping, and long-distance swimming.

But so far all these side effects have only been reported anecdotally by people using creatine. None of the scientific studies on creatine has proven a cause-and-effect connection between creatine and any of these symptoms. So, once again, we will have to wait for better studies to find out if there is any relationship.

Juhn and Tarnopolsky's 1998 study on the side effects of creatine supplements concluded as follows:

Creatine supplementation results in weight gain due to water retention, which may impede performance in mass-dependent activities such as running and swimming. Although short-term use (fewer than twenty-eight days) at recommended doses has not been shown to cause significant adverse effects, the studies on which this is based involved small numbers of subjects.

The researchers go on to say that future studies with larger groups of subjects are needed in order to evaluate long-term use of creatine on the kidneys, liver, and other organs. Recently, creatine has been found in many other body parts, including the brain, sex organs, and intestines. Although the amounts found there are small, we have no scientific evidence on how creatine may affect these organs over time. Caution is advised.

THE DEATHS OF THREE WRESTLERS

Creatine users got quite a scare in late 1997, when *USA Today* incorrectly reported that the FDA had issued a warning after the deaths of three college wrestlers who allegedly were using creatine. Although the FDA had issued no such warning, these deaths were investigated by the FDA, the Centers for Disease Control, and the NCAA, among others.

The three wrestlers, Joseph La Rosa of Wisconsin–La Crosse and Billy Saylor of Campbell University, who died in November of 1997, and Jeff Reese of the University of Michigan, who died in December of 1997, were wrestlers in training and trying to make their weights.

Creatine researcher Ray Sahelian, M.D., interviewed Reese's father, who said he has no evidence that his son ever used creatine supplements, and added that his son's college roommate had confirmed this. Dr. Sahelian further reported that Reese was trying to lose several pounds in one day and had not eaten or taken in any liquids for at least twenty-four hours.

Reese put on a rubber suit and exercised on a stationary bicycle in ninety-two-degree heat, in an effort to lose water weight very quickly, before collapsing.

In April of 1998 the FDA released information indicating that the wrestlers were trying to lose weight rapidly and may have been taking ephedrine, a substance intended to "burn fat," which is often combined with caffeine and aspirin. This combination, meant to suppress appetite, can have some dangerous side effects, including heart problems, especially if used in large amounts. The wrestlers may also have been using laxatives and diuretics to lose weight.

At that time a spokesman for the FDA exonerated creatine from responsibility in these unfortunate incidents, stating that "creatine does not appear to have been a major factor in the death of these wrestlers." And *USA Today* published a retraction of its incorrect story.

As tragic as these three deaths were, the subsequent reporting did a service to athletes using creatine, even though creatine use was not implicated in any way. It made them aware that they should know what they are doing when they use supplements or drugs, or carry out any conditioning programs designed to change their bodies. Without great care, moderation, common sense, and medical supervision, the results can be disastrous.

DRUG INTERACTIONS

None of the studies of creatine supplementation have shown any adverse drug interactions. But that doesn't mean they don't exist.

Again, to be safe, be sure to consult with your medical doctor to find out if there is any possibility that your use of creatine could interfere with any medication you might be taking.

It is known, however, that the drugs *cimetidine* (an antacid found in such medications as Tagamet), *trimethoprim* (used to treat urinary-tract infections and pneumonia), and *probenecid* (used to treat gout and as an adjunct in penicillin therapy) all interfere with secretion of creatinine in the kidneys.

It is also possible that combining creatine, especially in doses over 2 or 3 grams a day, with nonsteroidal anti-inflammatory drugs might put too much stress on the kidneys.

Discussing these concerns with your physician if you are using any prescription or over-the-counter medications is important before you make the decision to use creatine.

IF YOU'RE STILL GROWING

We've discussed how to buy and use creatine, how much to take, how often to take it, and whether or not to load or cycle.

But do these rules apply to everyone? No one knows for sure. And it's an area of tremendous controversy.

Should teenagers be using creatine? What about

younger children? Could it have an adverse effect on growth?

The young tend to think they're immortal and nothing can touch them. It's easy for them to ignore adult advice and do whatever they want to, because in most cases they won't experience the bad consequences for a very long time.

The fact is that, since there are no definitive long-term studies on creatine supplementation, no one can say for certain what effects it has on growth and development. Because of that, children and adolescents are at risk when they use creatine.

We have seen that taking creatine builds up stores in the muscle, often to maximum levels. Some experts think that this may signal the body to stop making its own creatine and that if supplement use continues, the mechanisms for making creatine may be damaged in some way.

Others say this is nonsense, and that as soon as people stop taking supplements, the body goes back to its former functions. Recent research seems to support this.

Creatine researcher Richard Kreider also points to the liability issue that is involved when people require or advocate the use of a substance that could later be proven dangerous.

"If there are side effects from long-term creatine supplementation," he notes, "an important issue will be the liability of coaches, trainers, universities, and athletic governing bodies who provide creatine to their athletes. Anyone advising athletes to take creatine should make it clear that side effects from long-term use cannot be completely ruled out, and that the athletes do not have to take the supplements."

Perhaps the best approach is to avoid using creatine until you attain full growth. But if you are a teenager and decide that you want to use it, your best bet is to use the lower doses for limited periods of time and then take a break of a few months before starting again. *But do not start until you discuss your creatine use with a qualified doctor and, most importantly, your parents.*

ETHICAL AND ATTITUDE CONSIDERATIONS

Apart from the possible physical dangers of using creatine, there could also be psychological dangers. And these do concern a lot of doctors, trainers, parents, teachers, and experts in sports medicine.

What message do people get when they use supplements to enhance their athletic abilities? And what do they think when they see famous pros such as Mark McGwire perform so well, knowing he is using them?

It is not so long ago that supplements of any kind were unheard of. People engaged in exercise and sport for the joy of it. Playing was fun. If you made pro, that was even better. You didn't make much money and had to get another job during the off-season to make ends meet, but you were still happy. You made it to the big leagues.

You worked hard to stay in shape and to be the best you could. You exercised, worked out with the team, learned the ins and outs of the game, and hoped you would get some kind of raise next year.

And then there were the guys who smoked, drank, stayed out all night, and got into all kinds of trouble. Staying in shape was definitely not one of their concerns.

But however you approached your sport, there's one thing you did not do: take performance-enhancing substances.

The arrival of sport supplements about thirty years ago was part of the revolution we have seen in the world of sports. Now, athletes are paid millions of dollars a year to play a game, and it's only a part-time job at that. They add on millions more with product endorsements. And before they get to the pros, the benefits roll in when they agree to go to a specific college. Scholarships, travel, media exposure, the works. Who wouldn't want it?

So today, the young athlete is getting a very clear message: if you want to have any chance at all of succeeding in the world of pro sports, with all its money, fame, and glamour, you need to bulk up with supplements. And the sooner you start, the better.

This is not a good message, nor is it correct.

And there has been a definite backlash against not only questionable or dangerous supplements, but all of them, creatine included.

This attitude is represented by Edward R. Laskowski, M.D., the codirector of the Sports Medicine Center at the Mayo Clinic in Rochester, Minnesota. In commenting on Mark McGwire's use of sports supplements, Dr. Laskowski says, "I think there's a danger that kids will think, *If I want to be like him, I'll need to take some-*

thing. I think we always tend to look for an external agent as a magic bullet, a magic pill that's going to help us perform. The truth is there isn't any."

Dr. Laskowski goes on to express his concern about coaches and players advocating the use of creatine. He notes that some young athletes feel bad when they find out that other players are using creatine and they aren't.

"In addition to the risk of long-term side effects," says Dr. Laskowski, "people may substitute it for proper training and think, *I can get away with practicing a little less because I'm taking creatine.*"

But think for a minute. It's true that Mark McGwire and Sammy Sosa both had incredible home-run years in 1998. But a huge number of baseball players are taking creatine. Why aren't they hitting sixty or seventy home runs too?

The answer is that creatine is only a supplement. It may provide a small edge for some, but overall, it's your natural ability and the gains you make from hard work that will enhance your sports performance. Whether or not you also use supplements should not be the focus of your concern. And they will never be able to turn an ordinary athlete into a superstar, no matter what.

Chapter 11

Creatine for Women

By now we all know that men and women are different in many ways, including the way their bodies function.

So just because creatine has certain effects in most men, that doesn't necessarily mean it will do exactly the same for women.

And, in fact, many women don't even want the same effects to begin with.

Yes, there are many female bodybuilders who work long and hard to build up their muscle size and definition.

There are, however, many more women athletes who don't really want increased muscle size, but do want greater endurance, more strength, better muscle tone, and less fatigue. So they're interested in creatine and many of them are taking it.

In reality the effects of creatine on muscles should be fairly similar for both sexes. We just don't know any of its effects on the things that are more specific to women, such as pregnancy or the menstrual cycle.

STUDIES

Nearly all the creatine studies to date have been done on men. So the findings and tentative conclusions we are discussing properly relate to men more than to women. Unfortunately, this is usually the case in the world of scientific study, but things are changing.

Many drugs, like Viagra, are tested and designed for men, but once they are approved, women are interested in trying them and the application seems obvious. Then, women's studies are initiated and women have to wait another few years to find out how the drugs work in their bodies.

So, with all the publicity about creatine, studies on its effects in women should not be long in coming.

HOW WOMEN RESPOND

Many women athletes have used creatine over the years. So while we don't have a lot of scientific data, we do have anecdotal evidence from what women have said about their results using this supplement.

You will remember that one of the main effects of creatine supplementation is to draw water into the muscles. And that a large part of the gain in muscle mass and hardness is due to this concentration of water.

Many women, who usually have smaller, less muscular bodies than men to begin with, have complained about feeling bloated when they use creatine.

Some creatine suppliers said that this was due to the characteristics of creatine in powder form, and they have promoted what they call a "stabilized" liquid crea-tine for women. They claim that using the supplement in this form will prevent women from experiencing the feelings of water retention and cramps that they some-times have with creatine powder.

These products often have other ingredients, includ-ing vitamins, ginseng, ginko, and digestive enzymes. You can check them out in the health-food store but you should do so only with caution. As with any supple-ment, you should research the ingredients and check with your health practitioner to ensure they are appro-priate for you.

DOSES

Most women who use creatine do well on lower doses. Products designed for women generally recom-mend an intake of between 2 and 2.5 grams a day, taken about a half hour or less before exercise.

Of course women, just like men, should experiment and see what works for them. Again, there will be a per-centage that will not respond to creatine and will feel no physical advantage from its use.

But when it works, creatine with exercise can pro-vide women with:

- increased energy for specific activities
- more lean mass
- less body fat
- greater muscle strength
- greater muscle definition
- less muscle fatigue

Again, we caution you that if you are a woman and want to use creatine, consult your doctor first. Just as with men, there may be reasons why it would not be wise for you to use it, and getting a medical professional's opinion before using this supplement is your safest bet. In the meantime we will wait for results of creatine studies comparing differences between use in men and women.

Chapter 12

Drug Use in Sports

There is little that competitive athletes won't do in order to excel in their sport. For the past thirty years or so this has unfortunately included taking drugs, many of them illegal and highly dangerous.

In quite a few cases in the past the drugs were provided by government, athletic associations, trainers, fellow players, or friends, often with the assurance "Everyone is taking them, don't worry," or "If you don't take them, you won't be able to compete against the others who are taking them. You won't have a chance."

Most of these athletes trusted their advisers, never giving it a second thought, while others felt it was only for a short time, just long enough to win, so it couldn't be so bad.

And then there are the athletes, like many in the former East Germany, who were given drugs and never even knew it.

The results have been disastrous, both medically and politically.

Some of the consequences of athletes using illegal drugs have included:

- serious health problems
- serious injuries
- death
- suspension from their sport
- banning from their sport
- disqualification from winning records or Olympic medals
- loss of public confidence in athletic competition

And everything in between. Every athlete in the world should now be aware of the dangers of these drugs. But their use continues, and many say it might even be growing. The lure of an Olympic gold medal, a championship ring, public adulation, college scholarships, and lucrative professional contracts for winners is simply too powerful to overcome a young competitor's concerns about possible side effects or getting caught.

But we can also say that this single-minded focus on peak performance has also led many athletes, who are unwilling to use these dangerous substances, to the much safer supplement creatine, now the most popular sports enhancer in history.

Even so, drug use continues to be a major issue in amateur and professional sports, and it is important to know something about the past and to examine the long-term connection that exists between sports and drug use. It's a problem that is still very much with us and one that should concern everyone involved with the sports world.

The problem can be seen quite clearly in the results of a recent poll of 198 current or aspiring United States Olympic athletes. They were given two different scenarios:

Scenario 1: The athletes were asked whether they would take a banned performance-enhancing substance if they were guaranteed to win and not get caught. A full 98 percent said they would take the drug.

Scenario 2: The athletes were asked if they would take the same undetectable substance if it would contribute to winning every competition for five years and then result in their death. More than 50 percent said yes, they would take the drug.

Pretty frightening, isn't it?

DANGEROUS DRUGS IN SPORTS

Although athletes have used many questionable drugs in order to enhance their performance, there are a few main categories that come up again and again:

• *Steroids:* Anabolic steroids are synthetic forms of the powerful male hormone testosterone. They are used to increase muscle strength and endurance and have been used for almost half a century. Legally available with a doctor's prescription, anabolic steroids are banned by organized sports. They have been linked to kidney and liver problems; cardiovascular damage; interference with the reproductive system, including sterility, shriveling of testicles, larger breasts in men, and smaller breasts in women; extreme aggressiveness; and premature death. We will go into more detail on steroids in the next chapter.

• *Testosterone:* Some athletes have used supplemental testosterone in order to accelerate muscle growth. Because people's natural levels vary, excess amounts can't always be traced by drug testing. But supplemental testosterone in people with normal levels can have some unwanted side effects, including shrinkage of the testicles and breast enlargement in men and masculinizing effects in women (beard growth and deepening of the voice, for example).

• *Human growth hormone (hGH):* There is no scientific proof that supplemental hGH improves athletic performance, but many athletes use it anyway because they say it gives them added energy. This substance, a chain of amino acids, controls the rate of skeletal and visceral growth in children and adolescents and, in adults, increases red-blood-cell mass and heart function. Taking supplemental growth hormone after full and natural growth has been attained is highly risky and can cause skeletal deformities by unnaturally increasing bone growth. It can also cause high blood pressure, heart problems, and potentially cancer.

• *Erythropoietin (EPO):* This hormone, used as a drug for treating anemia, works by increasing red blood cells in the blood. These added red blood cells improve an athlete's endurance and many competitors (especially cyclists) have illegally used EPO to enhance their endurance performance. Although it's almost impossible to detect its use in drug testing, EPO is still very dangerous. Because it thickens the blood, it has been linked to blood clots, which can cause strokes, heart attacks, and even death. In fact, multiple deaths have been reported.

• *Stimulants:* Amphetamines and other stimulants like caffeine and ephedrine help to keep competitors awake and energized. But the energy they provide is not true energy and can fool the body into not realizing it is actually tired, resulting in increased injuries and a sudden loss of strength when the drugs wear off. Certain stimulants, like ephedrine, can lead to arrhythmias, where the heart gets out of synch and starts beating too fast. The result can be a heart attack, stroke, or even death. They are detectable in drug tests, but there are also ways to mask them.

• *Other drugs:* There are quite a few other drugs that are commonly used to improve performance in various sports, including *narcotics,* medications that are used by athletes to deaden the pain from injuries and can lead to further and more serious injuries; *beta blockers* (heart medication designed to slow down the heartbeat), used by archers and shooters needing steady hands; *sodium bicarbonate,* which sprinters often use to prevent muscle fatigue; and *probenecid,* a masking agent used to prevent the detection of illegal drugs in testing.

THE OLYMPICS

It is the dream of practically every young athletic child to win an Olympic gold medal. Even a silver or bronze wouldn't be so bad. And countless parents share that dream.

To pursue it many sacrifices are made. Families spend enormous amounts of money on lessons and coaches. Sometimes one parent moves with the young athlete to live in the same location as a major coach, so the youngster can get the best training. And some children begin practicing for hours a day, from very early in the morning to very late at night, working on their sport, endeavoring to become the best, while simultaneously trying to keep up with their academic studies.

So when we see young people like figure skater Tara Lipinski win a gold medal at a very young age, we can be quite emotional. We know the hard work and sacrifice that have gone into making her the best in the world and we understand what a thrill it must be for her and her family to succeed so brilliantly.

An Olympic medal, of course, brings a lot more than public adulation. It also means a great deal of money for young athletes, many of whom are paid enormous sums for product endorsements and for their performances, especially after they become professionals.

But there is also a downside. The huge majority of young athletes do not succeed and never win medals. Many never get anywhere close to the Olympics. That could be due to many different factors, including:

- lack of natural ability
- inferior training and coaching

- insufficient money to continue training
- not enough hard work
- injuries
- bad luck
- personal problems

In other words, a lot can go wrong on the road to Olympic glory. So it's understandable that young athletes, their coaches, and their families are looking for ways to improve the odds.

Unfortunately, too many of them have settled on drugs, or "doping," as it's commonly called.

OLYMPIC DRUG TESTING

Gradually, over the years, the International Olympic Committee (IOC) claims that it has increased its drug-testing program, trying desperately to keep up with the huge number and variety of substances that competitors are putting into their bodies in order to better athletic performance.

But there are also many critics who see the situation differently. They believe that the IOC knows that Olympic competitors have been using illegal substances for a great number of years and they have tried to keep this information from the public in an effort to keep the all-important image of the Olympic games clean. In essence, these critics say, the IOC has been soft on drug use.

According to Charles Yesalis, an epidemiologist at Pennsylvania State University and an expert in the area of sports medicine, "The IOC has known about the drug epidemic in sport for the last forty years and has covered it up."

But whether they have done a good job or not, the IOC has nevertheless brought quite a few cases of illegal drug use to the public's attention, and has punished athletes who have been caught.

The IOC has prohibited the use of illegal drugs since 1967, when it wrote a medical code forbidding "substances belonging to prohibited classes of pharmacological agents and/or the use of prohibited methods."

Random drug testing became routine, and any Olympic competitor found to have prohibited substances in his or her body was thrown out of competition and had to return any medals that may have been won.

Unfortunately, increasingly sophisticated use of drugs and masking agents and apparently weak drug testing on the part of the Olympic Committee have led to the present situation, one that many critics deplore as riddled with illegal drug use.

People who know Olympic competition say that illegal drug use is rampant and very few athletes are ever caught. But for the few that have been caught, the results have sometimes been devastating.

Canadian track-and-field star Ben Johnson is probably one of the best-known cases. During the 1988 Summer Olympics in Seoul, Korea, Johnson tested positive for steroids. As a consequence Johnson's world records were removed and he was later banned from Olympic track-and-field sports for life.

But the most famous scandal began all the way back

in the 1970s, when the East German women's swimming team was widely suspected of illegal drug use. Winning eleven out of thirteen events at the Montreal Olympics in 1976, East German women swimmers continued to dominate these events until the 1988 games.

Then, after the fall of the Berlin Wall and the reunification of Germany, information began to surface confirming widespread drug use. It was revealed that the East Germans had a systematic drug-enhancement program for their athletes, beginning in the late 1960s. Supervised by their secret police (Stasi), steroids and other drugs were given to competitors as young as fourteen, often without their knowledge.

As a consequence of this information allegedly non–drug using athletes from other countries, who came in second or third to the East Germans, are now demanding that the IOC take back the East German medals and elevate the honest athletes into first or second place.

In addition, twenty or more years later, some of the East German athletes are now experiencing harmful side effects from the drugs they were given, such as sterility and physical deformities. One shot-put champion, Heidi Krieger, said that the massive doses of male hormones she was given eventually made her feel like a man and finally caused her to undergo a sex-change operation. She is now Andreas Krieger, a male.

Following the reunification of Germany many of the East German coaches got jobs coaching prospective Olympic athletes in China. The result? The Chinese women's team won twelve gold medals at the 1994

Rome World Championships, causing drug-use rumors to fly. To date a total of twenty-seven Chinese women swimmers have failed drug tests and been disqualified from competition. Does that mean the other members are not using illegal substances, or only that they have not yet been caught? While steroids are detectable, observers note that human growth hormone goes undetected with the type of testing now available. Once again the athletes and their medical staff may be staying one step ahead of the law.

FLORENCE GRIFFITH JOYNER

Questions about illegal drug use dogged the career of the late star sprinter Florence Griffith Joyner, who died in the summer of 1998 following an epileptic seizure that caused suffocation. While she always denied drug use, and no proof was ever found during her lifetime, many people familiar with the effects of illegal drugs continue to believe that they played a part in her success.

These critics point to the fact that Griffith Joyner's track performance was relatively undistinguished up to the time of the 1988 Olympic trials in Indianapolis. Suddenly, they say, her performance took off in a way that seemed impossible for someone undergoing normal training. The improvement was just too extreme, including the appearance of her muscles.

Winning three gold medals in the Seoul Olympics three months later, Griffith Joyner went on to have an outstanding track career for the next year. But after a total of only eight years she suddenly retired from the sport, prompting observers to note it was at the same time that the United States was about to begin a strong program of random drug testing.

On several occasions Griffith Joyner was accused of using human growth hormone, but no tests existed to detect it, so there was no way to verify whether the accusation was true. Whether she used any performance-enhancing drugs or not is unknown, but Griffith Joyner's sudden and dramatic sports improvement and her early, tragic death cannot help but make people wonder.

DRUG SCANDALS IN OTHER SPORTS

While the IOC endures withering criticism and may be pressured into strengthening its policies against illegal drug use, other sports are also looking at similar problems.

In fact, things have gotten so bad that the president of the German track-and-field association, Helmut Digel, has suggested wiping clean *all* track-and-field records at the end of 1999 and starting over, because the results are so tainted by rampant drug use.

It would take a separate book to detail all the cases of athletes who have been caught using illegal drugs. But here are a few of the better publicized.

In 1989 shot-put champion Randy Barnes was suspended from competition for two years after he tested positive for methyltestosterone, a synthetic male hormone that acts like testosterone. Following his suspension Barnes was again permitted to compete and won the 1996 Olympic gold medal in the shot put, only to be banned for life by the United States Track and Field organization when he tested positive for androstenedione ("andro," which we will discuss shortly).

In 1997 a participant in the Tour de France, the world's most famous bicycle race, was temporarily taken out of the race when he appeared to be using EPO following the results of a random drug test. (There is no specific test for EPO, but its use may be suspected when the red-blood-cell count is too high.) Erwan Menthéour, who said his high red-blood-cell count was due to dehydration brought on by diarrhea, later admitted that he had not only used EPO, but had also taken growth hormone, steroids, stimulants, and testosterone for several years in an effort to improve his cycling.

But the Tour de France almost ground to a halt the following year when a total of six teams had to withdraw from the competition and another team was thrown out because of suspected drug use.

In 1998 Czech tennis player Petr Korda stunned the sports world when he tested positive for steroids. At his appearance before the International Tennis Federation (ITF) several months later, they stripped him of his Wimbledon winnings and points, but decided not to suspend him. This decision provoked an outcry among many tennis professionals, who complained the ITF was soft on drugs and should suspend Korda.

They backed this up by pointing to the case of nineteen-year-old United States women's player Samantha Reeves, who in 1998 was kept on the tour after telling the ITF committee that she had the anabolic steroid nandrolone in her body because she had accidentally taken it in a diet supplement. In fact, the ITF has only suspended one steroid user in its history, the Spanish player Ignacio Truyrol, in 1996, even though many players say that drug use is quite common in the sport.

Cases of banned drug use have surfaced in soccer as well. More popular in Europe and other countries than in the U.S., soccer has millions of fans worldwide. Many were appalled to learn that Dr. Jérôme Malzac, a French physician, recently admitted that he had given the banned drug EPO to many soccer players.

There are many other cases like these affecting many other sports. In fact, most amateur and professional athletes can tell you stories about drug use gone out of control and about how difficult it is to compete without using drugs.

There appears to be an ongoing pattern at the highest levels, such as at the Olympics:

- athletes hear about performance-enhancing drugs and use them
- tests then become available that will reveal use of these drugs
- athletes switch to other drugs that can't yet be detected, or
- athletes use masking agents or other tricks to get around drug testing

And so drug use continues, with all its problems: unfair competition for the athletes, especially those who do not want to use drugs; unclean records for the books; and unwanted side effects that could cause health problems; and even premature death.

Why take these risks? Why run with the crowd without thinking for yourself? Why destroy your future for a few minutes of glory that may or may not ever come?

For fitness enthusiasts, exercise buffs, and serious competitors, there are safer alternatives. It's unfortunate that so many will have to find out the hard way.

Chapter 13

Anabolic Steroids

Maybe there was an excuse when they first became available. But not anymore. It's all cut and dried. **Do not use anabolic steroids.** They are dangerous, they can seriously harm you, and they even can kill you.

WHAT ARE STEROIDS?

Steroids are natural compounds or lipids that perform many useful functions in animals and humans. Steroids include cholesterol, sex hormones, and bile acids. They help the body digest fats, regulate internal salt and water balance, and foster the development of secondary sex characteristics. Certain types of steroids are used for a variety of medical conditions and are usually safe when used as intended.

There are two types of steroids in the body. *Anabolic* steroids build tissue up and *catabolic* steroids break things down, or block processes.

Catabolic steroids, such as prednisone, are frequently used by doctors to treat conditions including asthma, arthritis, low hormone levels, malnutrition, and certain cancers and skeletal disorders. They are not ergogenic and do not help to improve your strength.

ANABOLIC STEROIDS

Anabolic steroids are synthetic male hormones or androgens. Testosterone is the prototype anabolic steroid. The term *anabolic* means that these steroids affect tissue growth in the body. When used as medication, anabolic steroids rebuild tissue that has been damaged by illness or injury.

Their specific medical uses are rare, but include:

- treating certain rare forms of anemia
- treating certain types of breast cancer in women
- treating hereditary angioedema, a condition that causes swelling in various parts of the body
- treating hypogonadism (inborn low testosterone levels)
- helping patients gain weight after a serious illness, injury, or infection

In addition, recent studies have shown that two anabolic steroids in low doses can be useful for treating (1) patients who have been weakened by long-term kidney dialysis, and (2) patients who have been weakened by the HIV virus. So that under medical supervision and in moderation, anabolic steroids do have legitimate uses. For example, when anabolic steroids are used clinically, doses are usually low, in the 2-to-10-mg/day range.

There are different forms of anabolic steroids, including:

- nandrolone decanoate (injected, for anemia)
- nandrolone phenpropionate (injected, for some breast cancers)
- oxandrolone (tablets, for rebuilding tissue)
- oxymetholone (tablets, for certain anemias)
- stanozolol (tablets, for hereditary angioedema)

Brand names for these medications include Anadrol-50, Deca-Durabolin, Durabolin, Durabolin-50, Hybolin Decanoate, Hybolin-Improved, Kabolin, Oxandrin, and Winstrol.

Anabolic steroids can have serious side effects when combined with a large number of other drugs, so patients using them have to be certain their physicians are aware of all the medication they use, including over-the-counter preparations. For example, anabolic steroids can interact badly with acetaminophen, estrogen, and anticoagulants.

They can also be problematic for patients who have diabetes, enlarged prostate glands, kidney disease, liver disease, and some other medical conditions. In other words, anabolic steroids should only be used under the strictest medical supervision and only for the treatment of a specific illness, disease, or condition that warrants their use.

TESTOSTERONE

Anabolic steroids are very similar to testosterone. What does that mean?

As a natural part of the body male hormones are responsible for the development of many masculine characteristics, including deep voice, facial hair, and the male genitals. They are also protective of healthy bones and hearts, and are a vital component of a man's sex drive.

Women also have testosterone in their bodies (in smaller amounts than men), where it is an important component of their bone health and libido.

Under normal circumstances men make between 4 and 10 mg of testosterone per day and women make between 0.04 and 0.12 mg per day.

ANABOLIC STEROIDS IN SPORTS

The initial idea behind using supplements of anabolic steroids for athletes was to increase physical stamina and attain the kind of strength and power characteristic of very strong men.

Anabolic steroids, like creatine, seem to work best for anaerobic activities. They do not appear to have any real benefits for athletes who engage in aerobic sports, because they do not increase the rate of oxygen use in the body.

Steroid use generally results in weight gain, increased muscle size, extra power and endurance, and less muscle fatigue. Steroids also help the muscles to heal by markedly improving their recovery time. There is also a simultaneous loss of body fat.

These physical changes result in better overall performance for many athletes, especially those who need a great deal of physical strength for short-term, intense bouts of activity.

Taken in pills or injections, anabolic steroids have become commonplace in amateur and professional sports, despite persistent reports of their hazardous side effects.

WHO IS USING THEM?

Anabolic steroid use has been studied by many researchers, and their reports, along with much anecdotal evidence, indicate that steroid use covers a large segment of the population.

In a recent survey Charles Yesalis of the University of Pennsylvania found that steroid use among teenage girls had doubled over the past seven years. This amazing statistic was coupled with the fact that steroid use among boys in the same age group had declined.

Why? It seems that many of the boys have gotten the message that steroid use is not worth the danger involved, while a large number of girls are still focusing on the newly developing field of women's sports and are simply willing to do anything to succeed.

The Yesalis study estimates that there may be as many as 175,000 American girls between the ages of fourteen and eighteen who are using these illegal drugs. For the most part these girls are involved with sports in a very intense way, and some may be competing for the increasing number of college scholarships available in women's sports.

And then there is the plain old desire to win. At all costs. It can affect girls just as easily as boys. And, as Yesalis points out, these girls (like boys) think they can just take steroids for a while, build up their strength, get a scholarship, and then go off steroids to avoid detection in drug tests, which are far more common in college than in high school.

But even with this pattern of temporary or part-time use, the dangers of steroids remain. Girls are fooling themselves if they think otherwise.

As for boys, a study in the early 1990s revealed that approximately 6.5 percent of male high school seniors had used illegal anabolic steroids at least once. And there are many experts who think that figure is much too low, including Yesalis, who estimates the figure at up to 12 percent.

Overall, Yesalis estimates that there are about one million people in the United States (including the 175,000 girls and 375,000 boys from fourteen to eighteen) who have used or are currently using illegal steroids. They include not only professional and dedicated amateur athletes, but people from all walks of life who participate in sports or exercise and want to maximize their abilities. At present the most common users appear to be bodybuilders and recreational lifters.

People have a remarkable facility for ignoring the facts when it's convenient for them, especially in the area of drug use. The tendency to grab the short-term benefit and hope the long-term punishment never comes is very powerful indeed.

THE USE IS STAGGERING

According to recent survey findings reported by James E. Sturmi, M.D., of the Division of Sports Medicine at Ohio State University:

• More than one million Americans, including over 250,000 adolescents, have used anabolic steroids, either now or in the past.

• This figure includes between 5 and 11 percent of high school males and between .5 and 2.5 percent of high school females.

• More than 50 percent began taking steroids before the age of sixteen.

• More than one third of the students taking steroids are not involved in school sports activities.

• In one study 4 percent of children in seventh grade had used anabolic steroids.

• Between 5 and 14 percent of NCAA college athletes have used anabolic steroids.

• Approximately 15 percent of community weight trainers use anabolic steroids.

• An estimated 30 to 75 percent of professional bodybuilders use anabolic steroids.

In addition, these surveys showed that adolescent users of anabolic steroids are at risk for prolonged use; that most high school students were not afraid of the side effects; and that there is a strong connection between the use of anabolic steroids and other dangerous drugs.

THEY'RE ILLEGAL TOO

Not only are there health risks involved in the use of anabolic steroids, there are also risks of going to jail.

That message was brought home recently to the Dominican Republic immigrant community in Corona, New York, when a well-respected television evangelist was arrested as he tried to bring three jars containing three hundred illegal steroid pills into the United States after a visit back home.

His reason? He had purchased them in the Dominican Republic, where they are a popular remedy for children who don't eat enough. Calling them "appetite enhancers," Reverend Frank Almonte said that he bought the steroids from a pharmacy, hoping to help his twelve-year-old son gain weight. He said that he had no idea what they were or that they were illegal or dangerous.

Following his arrest, which could have ended with up to seven years in jail and deportation, Reverend Almonte's supporters rallied to his defense. And at a subsequent hearing, while over three thousand people stood outside the courthouse, prosecutors moved to drop the charges. Reverend Almonte agreed to take his son to a physician and to try to find a legal and safe way for the boy to solve his weight problem.

While certainly upsetting for the people involved, this case helped to highlight the problems of steroid use, especially in young people, and the dangers of getting caught breaking the law against their importation and illegal use.

In fact, steroids, under the control of the FDA, are illegal in every state unless they are obtained with a doctor's prescription. In addition, in some states, doctors must prove that steroids are being prescribed for a medical condition and not for athletic enhancement, or they can face prosecution. In California, for example, penalties for improper steroid use can bring up to a year in prison.

SOME BAD RESULTS

You've heard that anabolic steroids are dangerous and you should not take them under any circumstances (unless they are medically prescribed and necessary for some health condition), but what exactly do they do?

Here are some of the negative results of steroid use:

- shrinkage of testicles
- sterility
- stunted growth
- high blood pressure
- need to urinate frequently
- changes in libido
- hair loss
- tumor growth (cancer)
- tendency to violence
- heart disease
- liver failure
- foul body odor
- acne
- bloating
- sleep disturbances
- cysts
- high cholesterol levels

- male characteristics in women (including smaller breasts, deeper voices)
- female characteristics in men (including enlarged breasts, higher voices)
- cancer
- death

Are all these side effects permanent? Well, death is. And the masculinizing or feminizing characteristics usually are. But short-term use that causes minor side effects, such as acne or body odor, generally disappear when steroid use stops.

Why do men take on female characteristics and women take on male characteristics? It all has to do with the way steroids act in the body.

Normally, a man's body makes a supply of testosterone for his physical needs. But when supplements of steroids are taken, the body begins to halt its own production. The result is a shutting down of the masculinizing activities of the male body, resulting in shrinking testicles, enlarged breasts and nipples, lower sperm counts and possible sterility, and a higher-pitched voice.

For women the process is similar. There is a lessening of feminization and the development of such masculine characteristics as a deeper voice and the growth of facial hair, as well as disturbed menstrual cycles, enlargement of the clitoris, and shrinkage of the breasts.

Just as disturbing is the effect of possible stunted growth when steroids are taken by teenagers who are still growing. Boys and girls who were naturally going to be a certain height may find that they end up a few inches shorter as a result of steroid use. This effect is, of course, not reversible.

ROID RAGE AND MURDER

If you think that these physical side effects aren't quite enough to stop you from taking anabolic steroids, how about considering the psychological ones?

You've heard the term *roid rage* to describe the excessive anger that is characteristic of the personality changes in many people who are using steroids. Some of the psychological alterations they experience include the following:

- sudden, explosive anger
- extreme mood swings
- inappropriate aggressive behavior
- unreasonable loss of patience with others
- physical violence
- inability to accept rejection (or perceived rejection)
- hallucinations (hearing voices, for example)
- serious depression, sometimes leading to suicide
- criminal behavior, including murder

Experts have observed that the longer people use steroids, the harder it is for them to stop. In other words, they're addicted. And even when negative side effects begin to disrupt their lives, users can refuse to recognize the truth and continue on their path of self-destruction.

Can steroids really cause death? The answer is yes,

they can, although it is not always possible to directly connect the death with steroid use. For instance, one bodybuilder said that he got the AIDS virus by sharing a needle while injecting steroids. And in some cases young people have committed suicide while using steroids, and friends and family have insisted it was steroids that caused the personality changes leading to death.

But one of the most shocking side effects of steroid use has been its implication in murder. Not just one murder, but many. By adult bodybuilders who had used large amounts of steroids over a long period of time.

In a lengthy article entitled "The Muscle Murders," writer William Nack detailed the cases of several bodybuilders involved in steroid use and murder, for the magazine *Sports Illustrated.*

Probably the best known is Bertil Fox, a former Mr. Universe, who is currently in prison on the island of St. Kitts for the murder of his ex-girlfriend, Leyoca Browne, and her mother, Violet. Nack points out that this case is only one of the many instances of extreme violence that have been linked to steroid use. He says that some bodybuilders take as much as 3,000 mg of steroids each week, five hundred times the amount that the average man produces naturally. These huge intakes can quickly turn a calm, well-behaved man into one who is aggressive, violent, and out of control.

Another case cited by Nack is the murder of Kristy Ramsey, a steroid-using bodybuilder, by her former pairs partner Gordon Kimbrough. Now in prison in California, Kimbrough killed Ramsey after she confessed that she had engaged in sex with another man and no longer wanted to marry him. After the murder he tried to kill himself and immediately confessed when found the next day.

Yet another bodybuilder in California prison is John Riccardi, who killed his girlfriend, Connie Navarro, and her best friend, Sue Jory, in 1983. Nack describes these and other murders, detailing the killers' use of steroids and the psychological effect it had on them.

Can anyone prove that without steroids these murders would not have taken place? Probably not. Even so, there is plenty of evidence from people who knew these men that their personalities underwent dramatic changes following their regular massive use of steroids, and one of the main changes was increased violence.

There are perhaps thousands of different types of steroids out there in the marketplace, made by a variety of labs. Many of these products are impure and may even contain other toxic substances. If someone tries to tell you that the steroids they use or sell do not have bad side effects, or if you take them this way (which is called "stacking," meaning in combination with other substances), you will not be hurt, *do not believe them.*

If you're smart and if you want to stay healthy, physically and mentally, you will stay away from anabolic steroids—no matter what. Nothing is worth the risk.

Andro

When the word began to get around and athletes saw for themselves that anabolic steroids were not a very good idea, many of them started looking for a substitute, something that would have similar effects, but not as many dangers.

What too many of them found was androstenedione (also called "andro"), a substance that is just one small step away from testosterone. Maybe a little safer, but not by much.

MARK MCGWIRE, AGAIN

You remember that scene in Mark McGwire's locker room where reporters noticed that he had creatine and andro in his locker and McGwire freely admitted using both?

Well, there wasn't much fuss about the creatine. After all, it's being used by huge numbers of athletes and fitness enthusiasts, hasn't been banned by any pro sports organizations, has been widely studied, and seems to be pretty safe, at least for short-term use.

But there was quite an outcry over the andro.

Why? Because from everything we know, andro isn't safe. And because it has been banned by several powerful groups, including the National Football League, the National Collegiate Athletic Association (NCAA), and the International Olympic Committee (IOC).

In fact, when the information about McGwire's use of andro surfaced, baseball officials started to look at the situation and decided that permitting the use of andro in their sport might not be such a great idea, after all. So they began a formal study of the supplement, commissioning two Harvard medical researchers to determine exactly what andro does in the body. When the results are in, it is quite possible that baseball officials might also decide to ban andro.

But then if they do, what will happen to McGwire's home-run record? Will it be forever tainted and if so, is that what baseball wants to do with its public image?

So the situation presents a moral dilemma, in addition to its health and medical aspects, and it will be interesting to see what organized baseball (and the other sports that have no andro policy, such as hockey and basketball) decide to do.

In the meantime McGwire defended his use of andro, claiming that it is a natural substance and had done him no harm. "It's legal stuff," he told reporters, "sold over the counter." And so it is.

And that's exactly where hordes of people, many of

them under eighteen, are unfortunately rushing to buy their supplies, in an effort to emulate their hero and duplicate his feats.

MCGWIRE GIVES UP ANDRO

With all the outcry over his use of andro and the consequent upsurge in its sales, and use by young athletes, Mark McGwire apparently got the message—at least in part.

One day before he hit his five hundredth home run in August 1999, McGwire announced that he had stopped using andro at the start of the 1999 season.

Explaining that while he still believed it was safe for adults, McGwire admitted that andro is not good for children and he did not want them using it because of him.

"I always discouraged children from taking it," McGwire remarked, adding that he did not want people to think he was endorsing andro products.

A PRECURSOR TO TESTOSTERONE

Androstenedione is a natural hormone, produced in small amounts in the body by the adrenal glands. In the liver it is converted by enzymes into the male hormone testosterone. An average man produces about 3 mg of andro a day.

There are also small amounts of natural andro in meat and some plants. Andro's chemical structure is very similar to that of anabolic steroids. In fact, many say it *is* an anabolic steroid because it builds muscle tissue (anabolic) and is a steroid, or hormone. But others say that unlike steroids, andro is inactive when it enters the body, and requires the help of the liver in order to become anabolic.

Supplemental andro was developed by researchers in East Germany in the 1970s for use with athletes, including Olympic hopefuls. Its purpose was to boost muscle size, strength, and endurance, giving these sports contenders a competitive edge.

With greater-than-normal levels of testosterone athletes are often able to endure harder and longer training periods, and they can also perform better during actual games or competitions.

In the mid-1990s andro supplements became available in the United States market and sales took off. Manufacturers claimed that one 100 mg dose of andro would increase testosterone levels by up to 300 percent, a boost that would last about three hours. They also said that since it only lasted three hours, you would not see the same side effects as you would with anabolic steroids.

Unfortunately, there are few scientific studies on andro and most of the evidence about its supplemental use is anecdotal. And even if it does increase testosterone levels, there is no direct proof that it will improve your performance, especially when it comes to hitting a baseball. But there are many reports of undesirable effects in people who use it.

The only study on andro in a peer-reviewed scientific journal was published recently in the *Journal of the American Medical Association*. It noted that andro, in the doses recommended by the manufacturer, does *not* increase muscle strength and could potentially cause enlarged breasts, cancer, and heart disease.

In the study, conducted by Dr. Douglas S. King of Iowa State University, testosterone levels did not increase, but an increase was noted in the female hormone estrogen. This increased estrogen could potentially cause a drop in HDL, the good cholesterol (a 12-percent drop in HDL was found in this study), and cause an increased risk of enlarged breasts, heart disease, and pancreatic cancer.

In a journal editorial, it was recommended that the government consider removing androstenedione and its derivatives from the market.

WHAT'S WRONG WITH ANDRO

In a word, plenty.

Even the companies that market the supplement admit it.

For example, they tell you that women, and children under the age of eighteen, should not even use the product. Neither should anyone with diabetes, heart disease, enlargement of the prostate gland, or psychological problems.

The nationwide health-food chain General Nutrition Centers (GNC) has even refused to sell andro, banning it from their 3,700 stores in 1998. Explaining this decision, John Troup, GNC's vice president for scientific affairs, stated, "We're not yet satisfied with the safety of this product. We don't know its effect on the liver, cardiovascular system, or secondary sexual characteristics." And he added, "Clearly, no kids under eighteen should be ingesting this hormone at all."

But many other stores sell andro, usually in the form of pills or capsules, and sometimes in doses that are up to ten times higher than those considered safe. The cost for using andro? About fifty to ninety dollars a month.

Specifically, andro has been linked to the following problems:

- acne
- enlarged breasts in men
- heart problems
- liver problems
- personality disorders
- stunted growth
- loss of hair
- increased anger and violence
- shrinking of testicles
- sterility
- certain forms of cancer

Do these side effects sound familiar? That's right. They are almost the same list as the one for anabolic steroids. Taking andro is just like getting a smaller dose in your system, that's all.

WHAT HAPPENS IN THE BODY
Everyone seems to agree that a lot more research on andro is needed before we can know for certain exactly what it does and how.

But it does seem clear that only a portion of the supplemental andro even gets processed into testosterone.

First, it has to get into the bloodstream so it can get converted.

Andro manufacturers are aware of this problem and are trying to find ways to make a product that will be more effective. In the meantime people using andro may often take larger and larger amounts, in order to get the effects they are looking for.

And doing this only creates more problems. Because as testosterone levels in the body increase beyond normal levels due to the use of supplements, the body's own testosterone-producing mechanisms may begin to slow down. At that point it is possible that those functions of the body governed by natural testosterone can begin to fail.

That is why the use of steroids may cause a male's masculine characteristics to become feminized. Testicles shrink, breasts enlarge, and voices get higher, while in women the opposite can occur. Voices deepen, breasts get smaller, and the clitoris enlarges. And very often these changes cannot be reversed.

IF YOU TAKE ANDRO

Obviously, as long as andro is legal, it is difficult to stop people from taking it. You can just go into a store and buy it and if you're a pro, as long as your sport allows its use, there won't be any interference.

But it's still not a good idea.

If you are under the age of eighteen and still growing, your choice is simple: you should not use andro under any circumstances.

But if you are older and you insist on taking it, despite all the warnings and potentially dangerous side effects, then at least do so under the supervision of a doctor. And be sure to have your kidney and liver functions tested on a regular basis.

Don't exceed recommended doses and be on the lookout for any of the mentioned side effects. And don't use it for more than four to eight weeks at a time.

As with creatine and many other substances, individuals' responses to andro vary widely. In some people it doesn't seem to have any effect at all, while for others it seems to provide an immediate boost.

Experts say that athletes who are highly trained often experience the most benefits, possibly because their extreme rates of physical exercise have depleted testosterone stores.

But at this point it's not even certain that andro does much to help athletic performance. Even Mark McGwire has been quoted as saying that it doesn't help him to hit home runs, and he's probably right, or many others using andro would have similar home-run records. And Sammy Sosa, McGwire's nearest competitor in the 1998 home-run race, who hit sixty-six home runs for the season, does not use andro.

McGwire claimed that andro helped him with his endurance during workouts. From everything we know, you can probably get a similar effect, in a much safer way, simply by using creatine, that is, if you feel you need to take a supplement at all. At the very least you should wait until more long-term, detailed studies come out on andro before you consider using it.

And one final word: don't forget that if you get drug tested, you could test positive for andro and possibly risk being disqualified from your team or having your entire team disqualified. Is it really worth taking that risk?

Chapter 15

Other Muscle and Energy Supplements

Obviously, creatine, anabolic steroids, and andro are not the only supplements used by people devoted to fitness and sports.

Just walk into any health-food store, or check any supplement catalog, and you'll find so many it will make you dizzy.

How do you know what to take?

Some people solve the problem by staying "all natural" and not using any supplements at all. Instead, they rely on a good, well-balanced diet, regular exercise, and wholesome living. These athletes know they will not have to worry about any potential supplement side effects that may be discovered down the road.

Other athletes look at what the majority of people they know are doing, figuring the best will win out in the end. People like these probably take one multivitamin a day and maybe add some creatine for sports performance.

But other sports enthusiasts see things differently.

They are the people who throw themselves into every pursuit, and physical fitness is no exception.

They read countless books and articles about sports supplements, learning as much as they can. They try different substances, experimenting to see what works for them.

Many consult nutritionists, physicians, trainers, or their friends to find out which supplements improve athletic performance.

And how do they end up?

Well, some decide to take certain combinations of supplements on a regular basis because they seem to be the most effective. Others follow the advice given to them by experts and take what they recommend, no matter what the results. And still others do things at random, trying this and that, stopping this one and that one, with little method behind what they are doing.

The truth is that in the area of sport supplements, it is really difficult for the layperson to decide what works and what doesn't. And it seems that every day there are more new products to deal with. New formulas. New combinations. New discoveries.

But like creatine and andro there are certain supplements that keep coming up again and again. Some people have tried them and found they work. Or people have read the research and think they might work.

So if you're one of the people who have an interest in expanding your knowledge, and perhaps your menu of nutritional supplements, you may be interested in learning about some of the more frequently used muscle and energy supplements.

PROTEIN

Protein, made up of complex combinations of amino acids, is an essential part of every cell in our body. It is the basic material that makes up all our tissues and organs. Protein can be synthesized by plants, but not by animals. In other words, we depend on our dietary intake as our source of protein.

The reason is that of the twenty-three known amino acids, the body can only make fifteen. The remaining eight, also called "essential amino acids," must come from our diets.

The word *protein* derives from the Greek word *protos,* meaning "first." When most people think of protein, they think of meat, but there are many foods in our diet that are good sources of protein, including fish, chicken, turkey, eggs, milk, cheese, nuts, seeds, grains, and legumes.

The amount of protein we need each day is controversial. Some people say we need a lot, while others say that too much can be dangerous to our health. Some experts say that average people need about .9 gram of protein for each kilogram of body weight. Using this formula, someone weighing 200 (90.72 kg) pounds would need about 82 grams of protein a day, while someone weighing 135 pounds (61.23 kg) would need about 55 grams a day. Others say that protein should constitute about 15 percent of daily calories.

In fact, too little protein can result in such health problems as muscle weakness, stunting of growth, weight loss, fatigue, miscarriage, and a suppressed immune system.

But too much protein can also cause problems, such as stress on the kidneys, dehydration, and elevated levels of fat, cholesterol, and sodium, leading to weight gain.

Taking supplemental protein is also expensive. And amino acids, which we will discuss later, have the same potential side effects as protein.

Keeping the right amount of protein in your system helps to maintain your health. It affects virtually every function, including growth and metabolism (the process by which the body uses food for energy). Without sufficient protein we would not have healthy bones, teeth, skin, or nerves.

Because the body cannot store protein, you need to consume it every day, preferably with every meal. For those who eat meat, fish, and dairy products, this is not usually a problem. For strict vegetarians, who eat no animals or animal products, food must be carefully combined to provide all the needed amino acids in the correct proportions.

As a source of energy, protein can be converted into glucose, especially when supplies of carbohydrates and fats run low. Approximately one third of our protein is concentrated in the muscles. Normally, the standard amounts of protein would be sufficient for our needs. But there are times when our bodies need additional protein.

For example, pregnant and nursing mothers need more protein, since they are supplying it to the growing fetus. People recovering from surgery or serious illness also need more, because stress can deplete protein supplies. And people who exercise a lot also have elevated protein requirements.

Can supplemental protein, especially from a nonanimal source, help athletes and fitness enthusiasts? Some people think it can.

PROTEIN TO BUILD MUSCLE

Protein supplements have also been popular with bodybuilders, and recent studies show that weight lifters who work out for one to two hours a day need about twice as much protein as those who don't. How to get that extra protein?

A review of scientific studies suggests that in order to maintain the proper protein balance during short-term intense training and/or endurance training, athletes should ingest approximately 1.3 to 1.8 grams of protein per kilogram of body mass per day. Athletes who live in high altitudes may need up to 2.2 grams of protein per kilogram of body mass per day, according to a recent study. That is about twice the RDA for a normal adult.

Most of the time you can get enough protein quite easily through your regular diet, as most Americans do. But if you are a poor eater and you regularly engage in intense anaerobic activities, you might benefit from a protein supplement.

So how much protein do you actually need? Again, it is best to consult your personal physician, discuss your protein intake, and figure out what is best for your individual needs. The amount you decide on will depend largely on your diet, medical history, and exercise patterns.

WHEY PROTEIN

The protein supplement of choice for athletes who may need one is whey protein, and it is selling almost as well as creatine.

A trip to the health-food store will reveal protein supplements made in many different formulas. Some use animal proteins, derived from milk or eggs, and others use plant sources, derived from vegetables. But it is whey protein that is most popular with people looking to build muscle.

Whey is the watery or serum component of milk, which is separated from the thicker part, the curd, when cheese is made. Whey is very rich in essential amino acids, which make up as much as half of its content.

Studies of whey protein indicate that it may help build up the immune system when it is stressed by intense physical activity. Manufacturers recommend taking it (mixed with liquid) first thing in the morning to reenergize the body, and at night, before the fasting period during sleep.

Whey protein supplements come in several different forms, including:

- whey protein isolates (WPIs), the purest form, which is rather expensive because the fat, lactose, and sodium have been removed, leaving the protein in a purer form; and
- whey protein concentrate (WPC), less expensive, not as concentrated, and the form in most supplements. WPC gives you a lower

percentage of actual protein and a higher
percentage of fat, sodium, and lactose.

So if you buy, don't forget to read the product's label carefully in order to know what you are getting. Once again, we see a varying quality of protein products. Many times you can get the same protein benefits by drinking a milkshake, which can also give you added vitamins and nutrients.

Remember that whey protein is a supplement. That means it is intended to provide protein in addition to what you consume in your diet.

So if you are physically active, be sure to get the protein you need in your food throughout the day. And if you want to be even a little more precise, you could calculate your protein intake from food and only use as much of the supplement as you need to complete your daily protein requirement.

But the bottom line really is, do you even need a protein supplement to begin with?

If we look at the typical American diet today, we find that it is usually rich enough in protein so that supplements are not required to ensure good health. In fact, many people are consuming too much protein.

Clearly, the research notes that taking excess protein does *not* promote greater gains in strength or fat-free mass.

More recently, studies have suggested that pre- and postcarbohydrate and protein feedings may promote a more anabolic hormonal profile, helping the body resynthesize glycogen and/or hasten recovery from intense exercise. These changes may allow you to tolerate a greater degree of training over time.

However, these findings are only preliminary and the evidence is not clear as yet. What is clear is that if you need protein based on your diet/nutrition numbers and the intensity of your workouts, you should take it *before and after* you work out.

Do not be too quick to use whey protein. First, you and your medical professional should examine your nutritional needs and determine if it is really necessary.

If you become more conscious of your nutrition and dietary needs, you may not even need any protein supplements. So you should consider saving money and consult your doctor and a nutritionist, if necessary, to modify your food intake first.

AMINO ACIDS

Amino acids are carbon-based organic compounds that contain nitrogen, carbon, hydrogen, and oxygen. They make up protein and muscle. We have seen that the twenty-three amino acids that compose protein are also vital for the health of every part and every function of our bodies.

Fifteen of these amino acids can be made in the body, but the other eight must be obtained from our food. Each individual amino acid does its own unique job, and people use supplements of different amino acids for specific purposes. In some cases these supplements are used to enhance the building up of muscle and energy.

A few of the more popular amino acids used by athletes are the proposed anabolic amino acids, glutamine, alanine, and taurine, and the branched chain amino acids (BCAAs).

ANABOLIC AMINO ACIDS

Some people believe that certain amino acids, such as phenylalanine, arginine, ornithine, histidine, lysine, and methionine, may stimulate the release of growth hormone, insulin, and/or glucocorticoids (steroids), promoting an anabolic environment for the muscles. Some research suggests that large intravenous doses may increase your levels of growth hormone.

However, many others have been unable to replicate this in humans who take large oral doses. There is also little evidence that these supplements help reduce your body fat or make your muscles grow. Again, more research needs to be done, but anabolic amino acids do not presently look promising for enhancing your muscles.

BRANCHED CHAIN AMINO ACIDS (BCAAS)

Among athletes trying to build muscle, the branched chain amino acids (BCAAs) are favorites. They consist of the essential amino acids (the ones we must get from our food), isoleucine, leucine, and valine.

Why? Because these particular amino acids may:

- increase lean muscle tissue
- slow muscle breakdown

A considerable amount of research has been done on BCAAs recently. Theoretically, they may provide a nice environment for the muscles, helping to increase lean tissue and slow muscle breakdown. While several studies appear to support this, the research is really in its infancy and additional study is required.

More recent research suggests that BCAAs may be very important in regulating what scientists call "central fatigue." This term refers to the process where your brain signals your body that it is tired, even though your muscles might be able to keep on going.

Scientists believe that the ratio of BCAAs and tryptophan in the body affect the brain neurotransmitter called SHT. Increased SHT is proposed to cause fatigue, as well as a host of possible medical problems associated with exercise, including:

- overtraining syndrome
- anemia
- amenorrhea (loss of menstrual period in women)
- weight loss
- depression
- loss of appetite
- decreased work performance

Quite a list of changes for a few amino acids! Therefore, we have cause to be skeptical about whether there really is a cause and effect at work here.

Preliminary studies have shown no improvement in exercise performance or reduction in central fatigue. However, these studies were small and may not have been able to pick up minor differences. It is pretty difficult to measure psychological fatigue accurately, so more work is needed to find out the scientific facts.

If you use BCAAs, how much should you take? Studies indicate that about 10 to 20 grams a day, taken in two divided doses about a half hour before and a half hour after exercise, could help to provide a fuel source that will maintain muscle strength for greater periods of time.

If you want to calculate your optimum intake according to your body weight, you can take about .25 to .3 mg of BCCAs per kilogram of body weight. For example, a person weighing 200 pounds (90.72 kg) would take between 22 and 27 grams a day and a person weighing 135 pounds (61.23 kg) would take between 15 and 18 grams a day.

Remember to check with your doctor, perhaps see a sports nutritionist, and keep an eye on the current research.

GLUTAMINE

The nonessential amino acid glutamine, which the body can synthesize, is also one of the most favored nutritional supplements for athletes. In fact, some people classify glutamine as "conditionally nonessential" because in times of stress, stores can be depleted, requiring supplementation from food intake. Glutamine is said to help a variety of functions, including:

- bolstering the immune system
- enhancing muscle size
- repairing the digestive tract
- counteracting the ill effects of stress

- helping in recovery following surgery
- raising levels of growth hormone in the body

When it comes to stress, there are all kinds. Most of us immediately think of the negative types of stress: illness, overwork, injury, or worry over personal problems. But there are also positive kinds of stress, including stress on the body from a lot of exercise.

Stressing the body through physical activity depletes stores of essential nutrients, including amino acids. When these stores are used up and are not being replenished, the body gets them by breaking down tissue (including muscle). In the case of glutamine large stores are found in the muscles, so it is the muscles that will be broken down if the stressed body needs additional amounts.

For that reason people who are physically active may theoretically benefit from glutamine supplements.

Preliminary research suggests that taking glutamine supplements can prevent the decline of glutamine stores and can even increase levels in the muscle. But these studies showed *no* effect on performance or immune and muscle functions.

Available in powdered form, glutamine is a tasteless supplement that can be mixed with water or juice and taken in a similar way to the BCAAs, in two divided doses one half hour before and one half hour after exercise. In most products one teaspoon contains about 4.5 grams and the average cost is about ten to fifteen cents per gram.

Or, if you prefer, you can buy glutamine in capsule form. Each capsule contains 500 mg and the cost averages about ten dollars for a hundred capsules.

Some experts recommend an intake of 5 to 10 grams a day, while others recommend 15 to 20 grams a day. Or, if you prefer, you can calculate your dose by weight, giving yourself .35 grams for each kilogram of body weight. This method will give you a higher daily dose than 20 grams if you are bigger than average.

For example, if you weigh 125 pounds, you would take about 11 grams of glutamine a day and if you're 200 pounds, about 18 grams a day.

It is not a good idea to take your glutamine supplements with any acid-containing substances, since that will make it lose its effectiveness. For that reason many people take supplements on an empty stomach. The exception to this is if the glutamine supplement contains glutamine peptides; when they are present, these peptides protect the glutamine from acid destruction.

Glutamine also does not respond well to heat, so any dietary protein that is cooked will automatically lose some of its glutamine content. For that reason taking supplements might be a good way to ensure ample supplies.

Whether or not to use glutamine supplements is a very complex issue and it may take many years to find out precisely what is going on. The golden rule applies: more research, check with your doctor, consider seeing a sports nutritionist, and eat a healthy diet.

ALANINE

Combined with glutamine, this nonessential amino acid appears important when it comes to creating fuel for the muscles.

Although not as well known as glutamine, alanine is released from skeletal muscle when the body runs out of carbohydrates and needs additional energy. Traveling to the liver, alanine is an essential component in the production of glucose, which is then sent back to the muscles as fuel.

This type of cycle occurs frequently in athletes who engage in high-intensity, high-power activities, such as weight lifting.

There are not many studies on alanine, but it is used by many athletes, in combination with glutamine, to theoretically increase endurance and stamina. You should note that alanine is usually found in sufficient amounts in whey protein. But if you're not using whey protein and want to take a separate supplement, you might consider taking about 1 or 2 grams directly following exercise, so your depleted stores can be replenished.

TAURINE

Classified as a nonessential amino acid, taurine is theorized to provide physically active people with many benefits, including regulation of blood pressure, elimination of toxins, and stimulation of glucose uptake into the muscles. There are large amounts of taurine present in muscle tissue.

That means that taurine is probably an important

component in the production of energy. Like some other amino acids taurine can run low following heavy exercise, and supplies need to be replenished.

Both alanine and taurine have been poorly studied and cannot be recommended at this time. They are certainly not comparable in any way to creatine as an effective supplement for muscles.

DHEA

The hormone dehydroepiandrosterone (DHEA), which is produced mainly by the adrenal glands, has become one of the most popular sports nutrition supplements. Studies show that as we age, our body's capacity to produce DHEA falls dramatically, so it is especially popular with athletes over the age of thirty-five or forty. Some manufacturers even describe it as "the fountain of youth." However, there are very serious questions about its safety.

DHEA does have certain properties that may help to slow up the aging process. But there are insufficient studies to prove that taking DHEA supplements is entirely risk free.

DHEA is a hormone that may be converted to testosterone and estrogen in the system. Some studies have indicated that it may also help people to lose fat and gain muscle, especially those who do not exercise regularly, but so far there is no scientific proof that DHEA helps to build up muscles. Other claims for DHEA include increased energy and sexual drive, mood elevation, and prevention of diabetes and heart disease.

DHEA does have legitimate medical uses, however,

including treatment for people who have abnormally low levels of androgens (which can cause fatigue, depression, and a low sex drive). In addition, research is evolving that may show DHEA to be an effective adjunct treatment for certain medical conditions in older individuals, which are unrelated to athletic performance.

Potential side effects of supplemental DHEA can include:

- acne
- hair loss in men and women
- unwanted hair growth (particularly on the face) in women
- deepening of the voice in women
- breast enlargement in men
- irritability
- aggressiveness
- insomnia
- headaches
- heart palpitations
- elevated cholesterol levels
- damage to the liver
- higher risks of prostate and breast cancers

You will notice that many of these side effects resemble those of andro and steroids.

There is also concern that DHEA is being used as a recreational drug, with people ingesting large amounts in the hope of getting high and sexually turned on. Doing this, of course, can be extremely dangerous.

Since DHEA acts in a way that is similar to andro, some people who do not want to take andro use DHEA instead. Is it safer? We don't really know. But one thing is certain: *you should not take both substances at the same time.* And you should definitely have medical supervision if you take DHEA, because it is a powerful hormone that should not be used by everyone and could cause many different health problems if not carefully monitored.

Researcher Richard Kreider points out that there are no scientific studies that prove DHEA boosts testosterone, builds muscle mass, or increases strength. And Ray Sahelian recommends that anyone using DHEA supplements take no more than 5 mg a day, even though many manufacturers produce capsules or pills with up to 100 mg in each dose. So until convincing evidence of safety is proven, it is probably a good idea to avoid using DHEA supplements or to use them only in low doses and with the supervision of your doctor.

HMB

Beta-hydroxy-beta-methylbutyrate, or HMB, is another sports supplement that has become very popular. Athletes using it are responding to claims that it increases fat loss, builds up lean muscle mass, and boosts physical strength. It is also said to slow the breakdown of protein following strenuous exercise.

Some animal and human studies indicate that HMB supplements may slow the breakdown of muscle tissue and instead promote its growth.

HMB is sold in capsules and the recommended dose

is usually 10 to 12 grams a day in divided doses. Since HMB capsules are often no more than 250 mg each, that would mean taking forty or more capsules daily, at a cost of about five dollars per day.

At this point even HMB experts admit that they don't know how it works. So spending your money on taking it is very risky. There is some evidence that it may help promote muscle strength, since one study found that distance runners had less muscle damage and better leg strength after taking 3 grams of HMB a day as part of their training program than those on a placebo. And some people are even trying it in combination with creatine.

But there have also been recent studies showing no benefit at all from HMB. There is still a lot that we do not know at this time, especially regarding its safety, so it is wise to hold off on taking HMB until the scientific evidence is in.

MAGNESIUM

Although not a great deal is said about magnesium in sports literature, it is a very important mineral for athletes.

First of all, magnesium is necessary for the metabolism of calcium, vitamin C, sodium, potassium, and phosphorus. It is also important for the healthy functioning of muscles and nerves.

As a health supplement magnesium is proposed to work as a mood elevator, to promote healthy bones and teeth, and to treat indigestion. It is also recommended for people who drink large amounts of alcohol and women who take estrogen, since these two substances can deplete magnesium stores in the body. Food sources include seeds, nuts, citrus fruit, dark green vegetables, whole grains, figs, and apples.

The reason magnesium may be so important for athletes is its connection to the production of ATP. You recall how creatine acts to increase ATP and overall energy in the system. Well, magnesium is chemically bound to ATP and low levels of this mineral can theoretically result in muscle weakness, fatigue, cramping, and heart problems.

The recommended dietary allowance for magnesium is 350 mg a day, and there are many people who fail to get that much from the food they eat. The result is that many people are deficient in magnesium, and most of them don't know it. And, of course, those who get enough magnesium from their diets but are also very active can deplete their stores and need more.

The results of using magnesium so far have been controversial, but generally not supportive of its being ergogenic (helpful to performance). More research is needed before it can be recommended.

Your best bet, as usual, is to consult your physician and ask for tests that can measure your levels of magnesium and other minerals. If you decide to use it on your own, stick with low doses until more information is available.

VANADIUM
Another supplement used by people involved in fitness and sports is vanadium. This is a mineral that pre-

vents cholesterol formation in the blood vessels, helping to theoretically prevent cardiovascular disease. The best dietary source of vanadium is fish, where it is found most abundantly. But even when getting enough of this mineral from food, many sports enthusiasts are using vanadium supplements, in the form of vanadyl sulfate, because it has been reported to decrease the breakdown of muscle protein during workouts.

Producers of vanadyl sulfate, which has been used as a sports supplement since the late 1980s, claim it can "produce rock-hard muscle by lessening fatigue while reducing the breakdown of muscle protein for energy." Vanadyl sulfate products often contain other supplements as well, including chromium picolinate, L-carnitine, zinc, selenium, vitamin E, taurine, and manganese, which manufacturers claim increases the potency and effectiveness of their product.

Unfortunately, there are very few studies on vanadium and we simply don't know enough at this point to make judgments about its effect on the muscles in active people. A recent article suggested that it may even be toxic to mice in high doses. It is best to keep away from vanadium supplements until more is known. The risks far outweigh any potential benefits.

PYRUVATE

Researchers reporting on a study at the 1998 annual meeting of the American College of Sports Medicine revealed that there is evidence that pyruvate has properties that can help people lose fat and increase muscle size.

Pyruvate, a compound that acts in the body to break down carbohydrates and create energy, occurs naturally in the body. It seems to work better with exercise and has become a popular supplement for people who want to build lean muscle mass and enhance their physical endurance.

You should also be aware that most of the studies showing pyruvate's effectiveness did not involve trained athletes and were done with subjects who were overweight. It is quite possible, therefore, that the supplement had a more noticeable effect on these people than it would on someone who exercises regularly.

Pyruvate is available in capsules as either calcium pyruvate or sodium pyruvate, and studies indicate that taking between 6 and 10 grams a day in two divided doses can be effective for losing body fat and building lean muscle. But to do this is pretty expensive, costing up to ten dollars a day.

Manufacturers usually recommend lower doses, more in the range of 1 to 2 grams a day, but there is no real evidence that pyruvate at this level has any benefits. Research on pyruvate is in its infancy and it cannot be recommended at this time. It is safer and wiser to wait until more definitive information is available on this supplement before you decide whether or not you want to use it.

TRIBULUS TERRESTRIS

Athletes who don't want to use steroids or andro, but still want to boost their testosterone levels, have been using supplements of the herb *Tribulus terrestris*. The claim is that this substance will increase your body's production of luteinizing hormones, causing your body to produce more testosterone.

Luteinizing hormones are made in the pituitary gland, and in men they stimulate the development and function of the testes (where testosterone is produced). So the theory is that taking *Tribulus* will provide additional muscular strength and power. In fact, it has been used for some time in Europe by athletes, including Olympic competitors, and also as a folk remedy throughout the world. *Tribulus* is considered to alleviate infertility and impotence, elevate mood, function as a diuretic and antiseptic, and benefit people with liver, kidney, and cardiovascular problems.

Although *Tribulus terrestris* has been widely studied in Europe, there is little scientific data in this country and there is virtually no evidence that it enhances muscular development. Although some athletes have experimented by taking this herb in conjunction with DHEA and/or andro to mimic the effects of steroids, it is not something that can be recommended, due to the side effects of the former two and the unknown effects of *Tribulus*.

CHROMIUM PICOLINATE

Not so long ago chromium was being touted as an outstanding sports nutritional supplement for building lean muscle and losing body fat. In the form of chromium picolinate this mineral was widely used as a weight-loss product, but over the years results have been disappointing.

A trace mineral that works with insulin in the metabolism of sugar, chromium is important for normal growth, to keep blood pressure at optimum levels, and to regulate insulin. Its effect on insulin may make chromium an important mineral in the management of diabetes. In the diet it is found in such foods as meat, shellfish, poultry, beans, and brewer's yeast. Levels of chromium in the body lessen as you age.

Chromium was originally thought to be very safe. It was widely advertised and used as a weight-loss aid. Unfortunately, prolonged use or excessive doses have resulted in serious side effects such as anemia, chromosomal damage in animals (from picolinate), cognitive impairment, and interstitial nephritis (a kidney disorder).

It is generally thought that the average person needs between 100 and 200 mcg of chromium a day, and many people do not get that much from their diets. Even so, it is better to stay away from this supplement and, as with all substances that are not yet well researched, wait to get more scientific evidence on possible long-term side effects before you consider using it.

GBL

The story of GBL is the story of sports supplements gone wrong. A product that was promoted for building muscles, increasing sexual potency, and aiding sleep has turned out to be so dangerous that it has even caused death.

GBL, which is gamma butyrolactone, is a chemical that converts inside the body to gamma hydroxybutyrate

(GHB), a compound being tested for possible use in treating narcolepsy, a condition that causes comalike sleep.

The problem is that GBL has very dangerous side effects. Sold in some health-food stores and gyms, GBL was also available on the Internet under such commercial names as Gamma G, Remforce, and Revivarant. It is linked to the death of a woman who expired in her home shortly after taking it, and to such side effects as severe vomiting, seizures, fainting, and coma in others.

The FDA immediately intervened, asking all the companies producing GBL to stop selling it, all vendors to remove it from their shelves, and all consumers to discard or return it.

Several years ago, in fact, the FDA became aware that GBL was being used as a party drug and a number of women were hospitalized following incidents of date rape after they unknowingly took it. Now, with further problems, the FDA has announced that it considers GBL a drug, meaning that the agency has jurisdiction over its sale and is empowered to stop anyone from producing and selling it.

The problems with GBL, while extreme, are a warning to the many people who will take any touted muscle-enhancing substance without first checking it out. Don't do it. The price may well be much too high.

OTHER SUPPLEMENTS

Obviously, these are only a few of the more popular muscle- and energy-enhancing supplements. There are many others, as any visit to a health-food store or glance at a supplement catalog will tell you.

Are any of these products worthwhile? Did we skip one of your favorites, one that you are certain has helped your sport performance?

Some of these other supplements include chrysin, glandular extracts, potassium, saw palmetto, iron, and chitosan. New products are being developed all the time.

Then there are others, including choline, inositol, and boron, all common supplements that many people take. However, studies have shown that these substances are not ergogenic and they cannot be recommended for enhanced athletic performance.

So it's important to:

- stay informed
- read the literature
- talk to experts
- make sure you know what you're doing
- have continual medical supervision
- make sure what you're taking is what you really need
- immediately stop taking any supplements if you notice side effects, and consult your doctor
- remain conservative in your supplement use
- don't be a guinea pig and take any new supplements before they have been thoroughly tested over a period of years

From everything we know to this point, it is easy to say that creatine remains the sports supplement of choice because of its relative safety and effectiveness. It may not give you the same results as steroids or andro, but it also won't present the same dangers to your health.

By following a sensible program of good diet, exercise, and healthy living, you will find that you can still perform well in your sport and get the kind of rewards you are looking for without any supplements at all.

Chapter **16**

A Word to Parents

You would think that by now, most parents would be very much aware of the widespread use of drugs among teenagers and even younger children, and would be on the lookout for the first signs of trouble. But according to recent studies that is not the case.

When many of these parents grew up, the use of recreational drugs like marijuana seemed harmless, just a part of being young. They outgrew it and it didn't hurt them, many reason, so why worry about their children?

In addition, many of today's parents are working full time, sometimes commuting long distances to work, relying on baby-sitters, day care, after-school programs, or their older child's own self-care, when they are away from home. Sometimes parents spend so little time with their children, talking with them or really relating to them, that it's a wonder some of these children grow up as well as they do.

This message was brought home, once again, with the terrible shootings in Littleton, Colorado, in April

1999. The parents of one of the boys who killed their classmates, a teacher, and themselves, insisted that they were dismayed, that the young man who did this couldn't possibly be their child. Their son was a good, well-behaved, intelligent young man with a bright future ahead of him.

And the rest of the world looked on in judgment, saying, "What was wrong with you? Why didn't you see what was happening to your own child in your own home? Where were you?"

While the blame or cause for such problems can never lie completely with the parents, it is only natural to look first to the parents for answers—and to feel that if only they had done something different, this never would have happened. In some situations that may be the case.

TALKING ABOUT DRUGS

The Partnership for a Drug-Free America, a nonprofit corporation, recently published the results of a study of drug use among teenagers and younger children. The study also compared attitudes of parents and adolescents toward drugs. Their findings, involving almost seven thousand teenagers, over two thousand children from nine to twelve, and more than eight hundred parents, underline the gap that exists between adult and child.

For example, the study asked parents if they had talked to their children about drugs. Ninety-eight percent of the parents said they had. But when the researchers asked the children if their parents had discussed drug use with them, only 65 percent of the adolescents said yes. And only 27 percent said that their parents had taught them a great deal about the dangers of drugs.

If you think that telling your child over and over not to use drugs is a waste of time and will most likely have the opposite result, this study will make you think again. Because the researchers discovered that teenagers who heard a lot from their parents about the dangers of drug use were far less likely to use them.

In fact, 45 percent of the adolescents who said that their parents did not discuss drugs with them reported that they had used marijuana within the past year. Of those who said their parents had mentioned drugs at home, only one third had used marijuana. But of the group of teens who said their parents had told them a lot about the negative side of drug use, only 26 percent had used marijuana.

The study also examined the teens' use of crack cocaine, inhalants, and hallucinogens such as LSD, and found similar results. The more parents talked, the less their children used.

The study also revealed the different perceptions that exist between adult and child. When asked if they had ever tried marijuana, 42 percent of the teens said they had. But when the parents were asked if they thought their children might have tried marijuana, only 14 percent of the parents said it was a possibility.

If this study has any meaning, it is to alert parents to the importance of discussing the dangers of drugs with their children, openly, seriously, and frequently, and to be aware that you may not know everything about your child, even if you think you do.

DANGEROUS DRUGS

While the dietary supplement creatine appears to be safe within certain boundaries, there are other supplements and drugs that clearly are not. These are the substances that parents must watch for most carefully, since their use can have tragic results for their children.

We will not go into the use of illegal street drugs or inhalants, which many children use and which have been involved in quite a number of deaths, but we will have another look at drugs and supplements that may be used to enhance muscles and strength.

If your child is involved in sports and wants to be competitive, there will be great temptations to use these drugs and supplements. This is especially true of teenagers, but it has become a problem with some younger children as well.

STEROIDS

To the surprise of many the group that has shown the greatest recent surge in steroid use is adolescent girls.

Researcher Charles Yesalis of Pennsylvania State University found that between 4 and 12 percent of teenage boys admitted to using steroids at one time or another, but the real figure may be much higher. However, the rate of use among boys appears to be in decline.

When it comes to teenage girls, studies have found a rate of steroid use between .5 percent and 2.9 percent, lower than among boys. But the rate of use is increasing, and some of the users are as young as fourteen.

In fact, one study found that close to 40 percent of the teenagers who take steroids started taking them before the age of sixteen. How many of their parents know what they are doing? From all appearances far too few.

Who is most likely to be using steroids? It's hard to know, but if your child is involved in bodybuilding, weight lifting, football, wrestling, track and field (especially throwing events and sprinting), swimming, and cycling, the possibility of steroid use is probably greater.

We have already gone through the many dangerous side effects of steroid use, which include different forms of cancer, sterility, high blood pressure, shrinkage of the testicles, masculinization in women and feminization in men, stunting of growth, and a tendency toward violence.

But how can a parent tell if a child may be using steroids? What are some of the signs?

Although these effects could be the result of a number of causes, here are some of the more common signs of steroid use:

- rapid, unexplained weight gain
- a new case of acne or worsening acne
- hair loss
- a yellow tinge to the skin
- enlarged breasts in boys
- facial hair in girls
- swelling of the hands, feet, or head
- aggressive attitude and behavior

- sudden mood swings
- obsession with the body or distorted body image

If you suspect your child might be using steroids, what should you do?

Your first step should be to discuss your concerns directly with your child. This should not be done in an accusatory, argumentative way, with threats of punishments or the predetermination of guilt.

Instead, you should remain calm, let your child know that you suspect the use of steroids or some other substance, and ask if you are correct. You should then discuss some of the dangerous side effects of steroids and perhaps give your child some reading material on the subject.

Consult your doctor if you need help or assistance with this. Perhaps it would be a good idea to bring up the issue of drug use during your children's annual physical examination to get cleared for sports participation. In this way you can involve the doctor directly in the discussion.

It is important for your child to understand that not only are steroids *not* necessary for good athletic performance, they can also be a serious danger in terms of the health problems they can cause. You can offer your child a better program of performance enhancement through a healthy diet and well-designed workout program.

ANDRO

Since andro can act very much like anabolic steroids, it may not be possible for you to know which one your child is taking if you see some of the symptoms. You will simply have to ask and hope that your child tells you the truth.

Of course, andro is legal and readily available in many stores, while steroids are by prescription only, are banned in most sports, and are illegal in some areas if prescribed by physicians to enhance athletic performance.

Therefore, although illegal steroids are readily available on the street, it is more likely that your child may be using andro.

Should you be as concerned if your child is using andro and not steroids? Yes, you should. While children may not be breaking the law when they buy andro and ingest it, the dangerous side effects and health consequences remain.

It is also possible that your child is participating in school sports where there is random drug testing, and if so, a positive test for andro could mean serious trouble.

After you explain these dangers and discuss them with your child, don't be afraid to say that you do not want your child to use andro under any circumstances. If necessary, a talk with the family doctor or the team coach might also prove helpful.

CREATINE

Of all the supplements available to enhance athletic performance, creatine appears to be one of the safest when it is used as directed.

It is virtually impossible for parents to control every moment and every aspect of their children's lives. You can forbid your child to do something, but you can't completely prevent it. And peer pressure is very powerful. If everyone else on the team is using creatine, or if the coach indicates that it's all right, it might be difficult to stop your child from taking it.

With that said, our opinion is that under most circumstances your child should not be using creatine.

There are several reasons why, including the following:

- The long-term side effects are unknown.
- The effects on growing adolescent bodies are not known.
- There have been reports of many different side effects.
- It doesn't work for everybody.
- It isn't necessary for nonprofessional athletes.
- You can get the same or similar effects without supplements.

Although this book is largely about creatine, and although it appears to be one of the safest of the nutritional supplements used for muscle and strength enhancement, that does not mean that it can be recommended for everyone.

Of course, whether or not to use it is an individual decision, based on many different factors. But all things being equal, not even creatine can be recommended for use with children and teens who are still growing and who, in almost all cases, do not really need the extra edge it may possibly provide for highly competitive fully grown athletes.

ATTITUDES TOWARD SPORTS

While trying our best to be good parents, many of us inadvertently give our children the wrong message. We've already forgotten what it's like to be young and that the young often interpret things quite differently from adults.

We want to encourage our children, so we praise them. Your daughter wins a tennis game and you hug her and show her how pleased you are. Your son scores a winning touchdown in a football game and you throw a party to celebrate. Or your kids work out, their bodies look stronger and you're pleased, you encourage them to do even better.

Children have strong desires to please the important adults in their lives, parents and teachers especially. A casual word of approval can be taken in another way. For some children the message could be "I've made Mom and Dad happy and I've got to do everything I can to keep them happy, to make them love me and praise me even more."

This type of thinking in adolescents can sometimes become extreme and lead them to do unwise and dangerous things, including taking muscle-enhancing drugs.

What can you do about it?

One important thing is to focus on your own ideas about sports. Are you a very competitive person? Do you have the attitude that winning is everything and you have to do whatever you can in order to get that competitive edge?

If you do, you may be giving your child the wrong message. A message that could be harmful or even deadly.

A HEALTHY APPROACH TO SPORTS

As a parent you want what's best for your child. So it is worthwhile for you to take the time to examine your own attitudes toward sports and perhaps make some changes. And the sooner you do this the better, because many experts believe that the years from birth to three are the most powerful formative years in a child's life.

Sports should be fun. Especially for children. The main purpose of engaging in sports, whether competitive or not, should be to enjoy yourself. Young children's bodies are not fully developed, and they cannot do the same things that adults can. When their parents and coaches try to push them beyond their abilities, the fun often gets lost and sports becomes something else, something it should not be.

The goal should be to do your best. Again, this is something that often gets lost. Not all children are born with the same natural ability and not all children have the same drive to excel. It is really important for parents to remember this and to encourage their children to do the best they can and to praise them for their performance if they have tried hard, regardless of the results.

Everyone excels at something. Too many parents, especially fathers, focus solely on sports. Some of them may want their children to live out the athletic fantasies they never fulfilled or to reenact the successes they experienced when younger. Both of these goals are very unfair to your child. Every child is good at something, but not all children are outstanding in sports. It is a mistake to force your child to take part in sports when the desire isn't there, or to criticize and blame your child when his or her sports performance is not up to your standards. To do so could have a very damaging effect.

Sports teaches good physical health. When children take part in sports activities, they are often setting lifetime patterns for remaining physically active. They learn about how their bodies work, which helps them to do other physical activities, such as carpentry. Using supplements that may have harmful side effects can result in this important lesson being lost.

Sports teaches socialization. When children take part in organized sports, they learn a great deal about how to make friends, how to be both an individual and a team member, how to successfully handle winning and losing, and how to be a part of the larger community.

Sports is just one part of life. It's great if your child loves sports and enjoys playing or competing. But that has to come from your child, not from your desire to control or manipulate your child. A happy child is one who is well balanced and has many other interests in life besides sports. It is not a good idea to encourage your child to become obsessed about any one sport.

Remember love. The wonderful thing about a parent's love is that, ideally, it is unconditional. That means you love your child no matter what. And when it comes to sports, it will be regardless of whether your child performed well or not, or whether your child's team won or not. As long as children are playing because of their own desire to play, are enjoying the game, and are doing their best, you should not ask for anything more.

Children don't need supplements. Children should be encouraged to live as naturally as possible, to eat a wholesome, well-balanced diet, exercise, get plenty of rest and sleep, study, have friends, and have fun. In almost every case there is absolutely no need for a child to take any kind of sports supplement—it won't do anything much for sports performance and it could do a lot of harm.

If parents, from earliest childhood, teach their children to have fun when exercising or taking part in sports and if they don't get carried away by trying to have a child who outperforms other people's children, they have a good chance of raising a healthy child with a good attitude toward sports and toward life.

To summarize, here are some points for parents to keep in mind:

• Stay informed and find out all you can about sports supplements and drugs. Remember that new information is coming out all the time, so you must stay up to date.

• Monitor your child. Keep a close eye on your child's activities, physical condition, moods, and attitudes toward sports and toward life in general.

• Talk about drugs, supplements, and the meaning

of sports in your child's life. Do this frequently. Don't preach or make judgments, just be certain your child understands your views and the reasons behind them, and how you feel about the use of muscle and energy enhancers. One good time to discuss these things is during your child's annual physical exam.

• Take a conservative approach. When it comes to supplements or drugs, the rule should be "less is better." Ideally, your child should not use them, but if there is some very good reason for their use, creatine, in limited amounts, is one of your safest bets.

• Make decisions about supplement or drug use in coordination with your child, your child's doctor, and any other health or sports professionals you trust.

• If your child is a professional athlete or a serious Olympic contender, there may be a place for creatine use. Again, this should be worked out with professional advice.

Chapter 17

Before You Take Creatine

It is hard to sift through all the material on the benefits of creatine as well as the possible risks involved, and then make a clear decision.

In order to help you make your decision, you can try the following self-administered quiz:

1. Are you at least eighteen years old?
2. Do you regularly engage in anaerobic sports, that is, most days of the week, either year-round or during your sport's season?
3. Does your sport involve short-term, intense bouts of activity, such as throwing the javelin, hitting a baseball, or sprinting a short distance?
4. Do you eat a well-balanced diet?
5. Do you get all the rest and sleep you need?
6. Are you free from kidney disease or a family history of kidney disease?

7. Do you have an annual physical exam?

8. Are you generally healthy?

9. Are you underweight or do you want to gain some weight?

10. Do you drink plenty of fluids every day, at least eight eight-ounce glasses or more?

11. Are you a reliable person, and once you undertake a program, do you stick to it without failure?

12. Can you afford to take supplements on a regular basis?

13. Are you willing to take the time to do some research to find out more about supplements and which one might be the best for you?

14. Do you have a coach or trainer who is well informed on supplements and whose advice you respect?

15. If you decide to use supplements, do you have a well-informed health-care professional who can regularly monitor your progress?

16. Have you clarified and written down your goals for using supplements and do they seem reasonable to you?

17. Have you thought about what sport means to you and what place it plays in your total life?

18. Are you a professional athlete, an Olympic hopeful, or someone who takes part in regular anaerobic sports contests and competitions?

19. Do you see supplements as only one small part of your total sports program?

20. If supplements do not work for you, will

you still enjoy your sport and feel good about yourself?

If you answer yes to most of these questions, then you can probably give serious consideration to using creatine. This does not mean you *should* use it, only that you are a viable candidate.

Chapter 18

Questions and Answers About Muscle-Enhancing Sports Supplements

Even when you do your homework and keep up-to-date on all the available facts, many questions remain. Here are some frequently asked questions about creatine and other muscle-enhancing sports supplements, with answers provided by Dr. Monaco.

Q: I live in a small town and my doctor doesn't know anything about creatine, andro, or any other sports supplements. What should I do?

A: There are many health-care providers who are familiar with sports supplements, including nutritionists. Some of them are specialized sports nutritionists and may belong to the American Dietetic Association (ADA). You can also contact your local university, college, or academic health center and ask for a sports-medicine doctor. If there is no one at the college or university who has this knowledge, you can probably get a referral to someone who does. Doctors who specialize in primary-care sports medicine should also be of great help.

Q: I eat a lot of meat and animal products. Does that mean I need less creatine?

A: We know that vegetarians usually have slightly less creatine stores than nonvegetarians. However, the body—even in vegetarians—tends to make more creatine when it is needed. In the amounts that we are talking about for high-intensity sports activity, you would require so much food containing creatine that you could not get it through your diet alone.

In addition, even if you do need less creatine, there is no scientific way to determine the exact amount you need, partly because there is such a variable range in how much people have to begin with. So there is no easy way to determine your most effective dose. It's best to stick with a standard dose that has been established through studies, rather than play around with half a gram less, for instance. So even though you may need a little less, since there's no effective way to determine it, it is wiser to stay with the protocols that have been shown to work.

Q: Is it true that if you use creatine you won't get so many sports injuries?

A: There is no literature to suggest that creatine will reduce sports injuries. There is anecdotal evidence to suggest that creatine may actually cause an *increase* in muscle injuries. However, no studies have proven this yet. But some people believe that the rapid muscular expansion that can occur with creatine may stress the tendons, ligaments, bones, and joints so much that they have not had a chance to fully adapt. Then, if you are stronger but your tendons haven't had the time to catch up with your muscles, and you go out and do activities, you may end up with more tendinitis, strains, and sprains.

The evidence that this might occur is theoretical right now. Since we don't have any scientific proof of it so far, we will just have to wait and see what happens over the next few years to determine if increased injury patterns are connected with the use of creatine.

Q: I'm a bodybuilder and I used steroids for five years. I stopped when I started to get some bad side effects. Is there any way to reverse these changes, which include a higher voice and smaller testicles?

A: Many of the effects of steroids are irreversible. There are some available treatments, including surgery and the use of hormones, to counteract these problems in men. However, these treatments could themselves cause other undesirable side effects. I advise you to consult with an endocrinologist, who is a specialist in this area, and get professional advice regarding your individual condition.

Q: I took creatine for a month and nothing happened. I do weight training and play basketball and jog. Why didn't it work for me, and is there something else that will work?

A: Certain people are nonresponders and do not experience any benefits from using creatine. You should also ask yourself why you tried creatine. If you play recreational basketball and jog, you are not likely to see any real clinical benefits from taking creatine, since you are engaging mainly in aerobic activities. So you should reevaluate why you want to use it and what you hope to get out of it.

Another thing you can do is check the dosage and see if you were taking enough for your body-weight/body-fat ratio. Finally, if you do not gain any weight from using creatine, especially following the initial loading period, you may be one of the approximately 20 percent of people who, for one reason or another, do not respond to the use of creatine supplements.

Q: I have seen creatine candy bars and chewing gum. Are these products any good?

A: The amount of creatine that you get from candy bars and chewing gum is so small that it is really not worth the money you're paying for it. You would be much better off staying with the powder form and taking your regular dosage that way. You can use these products if you want to, but they are probably not cost effective in terms of delivering creatine.

Q: I've been told that creatine is not good for aerobic activities. I'm a marathon runner. If I take it, could it help me in any way?

A: Creatine does not show benefits for aerobic activity. But it may be helpful in certain strength phases of your training. You should discuss this with your sports physician or trainer to decide if it might have a place in your program.

Q: Is there a problem combining creatine with other bodybuilding supplements like DHEA or HMB?

A: We don't know if there are any reactions from combining creatine with other supplements. That aspect of creatine has not been well studied as yet. I would advise you to stick to taking just pure creatine and not combine it with other supplements.

HMB may be of some benefit in building muscle, but I think it needs to be looked at individually. So far it has not been very well studied. There have been two studies indicating that HMB may be of some benefit, but they were done with nonathletes. More recent studies showed poor results. So I would say that each supplement needs to be looked at on an individual basis and that most scientific studies do not look at combining supplements. I think that rather than combining supplements at this time when the effects remain unknown, you should stick with individual supplements in recommended amounts until further testing is done.

Q: How much liquid do I need to drink every day when I'm on creatine?

A: You should consume a few glasses more than the normal recommended amount, which is eight eight-ounce glasses per day. One formula recommends that in addition to these sixty-four daily ounces, you add one eight-ounce glass of water for every fifteen minutes you exercise. When you use creatine, you do need additional fluid or you risk becoming dehydrated.

Q: I'm in high school and really can't afford the cost of creatine. Is there something cheaper that would work as well?

A: You can try eating a normal amount of meat in your diet, but it has to be balanced with all the other foods you need, including fruit, vegetables, grains, and dairy. If you are interested in building muscle and strength, nothing replaces hard work. It's that simple.

Q: A lot of supplement packages say they're "all natural." Does that mean anything?

A: *All natural* does not mean anything. It is just a phrase used to sell a product. If you want to know what's in a product, read the label carefully and, if necessary, contact the manufacturer for additional information.

Q: I have two children, ages fifteen and nine. Is it safe for them to use creatine?

A: Based on what we know about creatine and how it works in the body, it appears that there will be little risk for adolescents taking it. Currently, we know that it does not work like a hormone, so it should not pose any long-term risk for younger children, but there are no studies much longer than two years at this point, so it is safer if they do not use it.

What we should emphasize is that using creatine is very similar to eating a natural substance. You're just taking larger doses, so it should not be a problem. It is similar to carbohydrate loading on a daily basis, which would not pose any long-term problems.

But even though creatine is well studied, most of the studies are on people who are eighteen years of age and older, so to be safe, you should be cautious in using it with younger children. Although we don't anticipate that the effect of creatine would be different on adults and teenagers, at this point we do not know for certain.

So for your fifteen-year-old I would recommend using it with caution if you think it serves an appropriate purpose. For the nine-year-old, I think it is best at that age to develop skills in the sport you choose and to learn appropriate training techniques and habits, rather than look for an increase through a synthetic substance.

There is also the ethical question of using creatine with children. Do we want to teach younger children to rely on a supplement rather than natural training? So I tend not to recommend it for children under eighteen, especially since the benefits may not even be noticeable on the playing field.

In the event that you decide your children should use creatine, be sure to monitor them closely and to have appropriate medical supervision.

Q: Do creatine and andro show up on drug testing?
A: Andro can show up on drug testing when you look for the ratio of testosterone to epitestosterone. But creatine cannot be tested for at this time. The governing sports bodies have talked about testing for creatine, so there may be some research going on to try to develop ways to detect it. But creatine is a natural substance and it may be difficult to develop an effective test for it.

Q: I'm just starting to work out after years of being a couch potato. Should I start using creatine now or should I wait until I've built up some muscle through exercise?

A: It's great that you are starting to exercise and I would encourage you to continue. People who start on an exercise program should look at what they want to get out of it and they should make gradual changes in their program as they progress. For someone like you, who is just starting out and who is a recreational athlete, it is probably not worthwhile for you to take creatine. You are going to get a lot of benefits just from working out and you really don't have any need for supplements at this time.

Q: Do you really need to take whey protein if you have a high-protein diet?
A: I am not a big fan of whey protein. From everything I understand now and from the literature, whey protein is largely a gimmick. It may be of some benefit to super-bodybuilders, but 99.9 percent of people get too much protein in their diets anyway, so I am not very big on promoting protein supplements. However, whey protein can be of benefit for a very small segment of people.

Q: I have always been very skinny and I cannot gain weight, no matter what I try. Somebody told me creatine helps you gain weight. Can I use it just for that and if so, how do I do it?
A: Some people want to gain weight. Some of them are eighteen or nineteen, have always been very thin, and don't seem to gain weight through eating more. For people like this, creatine can be used for weight gain. I have seen it work in many cases. The usual weight gain

is anywhere from two to seven pounds. But the risks and benefits need to be evaluated. If you decide to use creatine for gaining weight, it should be done only along with an appropriate healthy diet and a resistance-training strength program.

Q: If I stop using creatine, will that reverse the muscle mass I've gained?

A: It will not reverse the muscle mass that you built up naturally through lifting or resistance-training activities. However, once you stop using creatine, the amount of creatine within your muscles will go down and you may lose some volume within these muscles. You may notice this in your resistance-training exercises. The level usually drops anywhere between two and six weeks after you stop using creatine. However, you never lose that hard work you've done. That does not disappear because you are not using a supplement anymore, as long as you continue working out. If you stop working out, though, you will have some natural degradation of muscle mass. This also occurs naturally with the aging process.

Q: My kidneys are fine, but there is a history of kidney disease in my family. Is it safe for me to use creatine?

A: Our current knowledge does not suggest that creatine poses an additional stress to the kidneys in the doses that are recommended. However, you should remember that most creatine studies do not extend beyond a two-year period. Because of that and the fact that there may be long-term information we do not yet have, we recommend that anyone with an individual or a family history of kidney disease not use creatine, to be on the safe side.

There have also been a few cases that indicate there may be a problem. For example, there was a case published in the medical journal *Lancet,* about someone who was on kidney dialysis for a while. Then, when he was off dialysis, he started using creatine. After a short period of time he had to go back on dialysis. But the report did not prove a direct cause-and-effect between the use of creatine and the need for dialysis, so the argument did not hold up well.

My conclusion is that anyone who has or may have underlying kidney disease should stay away from creatine until there are more long-term studies out that prove it is not a danger.

Q: Do I need any lab tests before I take creatine or other sports supplements?
A: Most of the people using sports supplements have not had any lab tests and most of them do well. However, it would be prudent to make sure that your kidneys are functioning normally and that you are not having any health problems before you begin long-term use of any supplement.

I would recommend that you sit down with a healthcare professional and look at your total health. Why do you want to take a supplement and what are you looking to get out of it? Do you have any medical problems that might get worse if you use supplements?

And I would recommend that you consider a normal chemistry panel, which will look at your lipids, your cholesterol, and your liver function. You could also get a serum creatinine or blood creatinine test and a blood/urea/nitrogen (BUN) test, which are included in a basic chemistry panel.

If you are considering long-term use, or if you are an adolescent, it is really a good idea to see a doctor and have normal blood tests and make sure there aren't any underlying problems that you don't know you have. You can use that occasion to talk to your physician about why you want to use creatine, how you plan to use it, and what you expect to gain from it.

Q: I want to find out my vitamin and mineral levels. Is a hair test a good way to find out?

A: Hair tests are not reliable. But blood tests are not reliable for a lot of vitamins and minerals either. The amounts of individual vitamins and minerals in your body change constantly and tests are not always able to calculate the exact amounts.

We can test for some vitamins, like vitamin B_{12} or folate, by doing blood tests, which are pretty accurate. Hair tests give results that, even if accurate, are two or three months old, so they don't necessarily relate to your current vitamin and mineral levels.

If you are concerned about your vitamin and mineral levels, your best bet is to discuss this with your doctor, who may be able to get you some information from blood tests.

Q: I've been using creatine for a few weeks and have had some cramps. Should I consult my doctor?

A: Definitely. Anyone who has side effects from creatine or any other supplement should be examined by a physician. If someone takes creatine and begins to cramp a lot, I do blood tests and if I see a lot of changes, I take the person off the supplement.

Sometimes we don't know if these changes are due to creatine or not. They could just be a result of exercise. We know that exercise alone builds body mass and causes elevated creatinine levels in the serum, so when we find higher creatinine levels, we can't determine if it's a result of taking creatine supplements or from additional physical activity. But if the numbers get really high, we just take the athlete off the supplements, to be safe. It's not something we want to fool around with.

Q: I'm in training and try to take creatine every day. But what will happen if I miss a day or two?

A: Nothing will happen, but your creatine levels may drop off and you should resume your normal dose as soon as you can. If you keep missing a day or two here and there, you may end up with having too low a dose to see benefits. If that happens, you should reevaluate why you are taking it and how strong your commitment is to the benefits you are trying to obtain.

One of the big problems we find with young people is that they load, then they miss four or five days because they go away or something, then they take creatine, then they forget, and so on. So you can't really tell if it's going to help them or not. We encourage people, especially early on, to give creatine a true trial and see what happens when you maximize your levels, which means taking it on a regular basis and not missing any days. Otherwise, you're just spending a lot of money and not getting any true benefits from it.

Q: I'm a bodybuilder and I'm looking for more muscle definition. Will creatine do this for me?

A: Creatine does cause muscle hypertrophy (the enlargement or growth of an organ or part due to an increase in the size of its constituent cells) in the people who respond to it, so it can enhance the look of your muscles. But don't forget that you need to exercise and follow your program in order to get good results.

Q: I'm sixty-two years old, had a stroke two years ago, and have partial muscle paralysis on my right side. I work out regularly and want to know if I can use creatine.

A: There should be no problems with your using creatine, provided you have no other health problems. You should discuss your desire to use creatine with your doctor and ask if it would interfere with any medication you are using or any medical condition you may have. As a rule older people with medical problems should involve their primary physicians before they consider taking a course of supplements such as creatine. If you decide to use it, make sure your doctor monitors you for benefits and risks.

Q: What is the maximum amount of creatine you can use?

A: We don't know the answer to that question. We do know that there is a saturation level within the body and once you reach that point, any extra creatine will have no benefit at all. We can generalize that taking more than about 25 grams of creatine a day, depending on your size and weight, is probably not going to be of benefit.

You can check the information on loading and maintenance according to your weight and take either that amount or the standard recommended daily doses to be safe. Anything above the saturation point will not provide any additional benefits.

Q: I'm concerned about the possible long-term effects of creatine. Has it been checked out as thoroughly as prescription drugs?

A: Creatine has been around a long time. Some investigations began in the 1920s and it has been used as a supplement since the 1960s, especially with a large number of athletes in Eastern Europe. Since the early 1990s we have had at least two hundred papers on creatine, so it has been very well studied. But not as well as many prescription drugs.

The pharmaceutical companies usually study larger numbers of people and their studies are more controlled, so the results are more scientifically rigorous. Most of the creatine studies have been on small numbers of people, increasing the chance that error in the research may be affecting the results.

On the other hand, many prescription drugs have been FDA-approved and in the first year of sale have been found to have serious side effects and are sometimes withdrawn or reformulated. Millions of people have used creatine over the past few years and we haven't seen anything substantial reported in the literature on bad side effects. So in one sense the unscientific laboratory of daily use has substantiated that creatine has held up very well, so far.

Q: Can the loading phase be dangerous because of the large amounts you are taking? Can they be some kind of shock to the body?

A: It does not appear to add any significant risk to go through a loading phase with creatine. Some people think that it down-regulates the creatine receptors, so your body does not make as much endogenously. But in the limited research that is out there, there is support that over time, creatine levels in the body will return to normal.

These studies, however, are short term and we do not have data from a three- or four-year period. Nonetheless, creatine loading may create a stress across the kidneys, so it is my recommendation that you avoid the loading phase at times when you are under a lot of heat stress or you are exercising in hot, humid weather. If you have the luxury of time (approximately one month) to see results, I recommend you avoid loading and use the regular maintenance dose.

If you use a loading phase, you should make sure that your fluid intake is optimal. You should also avoid the use of any nephrotoxic (dangerous to the kidneys) drugs while loading, so do not take Advil, Aleve, or other nonsteroidal over-the-counter products that can cause problems.

Q: I'm a long-distance runner and have been told that creatine will not do much for me. I want better strength and endurance. Which supplements could benefit me?

A: You are correct that creatine has not been shown to be beneficial for long-distance aerobic activities. However, there may be certain times in your training periods when you're trying to enhance strength and creatine could be useful. There is also some preliminary work suggesting that taking creatine may enhance the uptake of glycogen into the muscles. Glycogen is known to help long-distance aerobic activity, and it is a significant benefit. So keep posted on the evolving literature in this regard.

In reference to other supplements the main thing is really going to be glycogen replacement. Glycogen is a natural substance that you get from food, like creatine, and it can be useful in more concentrated supplemental form. There are a few other supplements that may be helpful, including caffeine, which has been shown to be of some benefit at higher doses, but I would not suggest experimenting with it at this time.

Q: Is it better to use just plain creatine powder or to use one of the products that have other ingredients?

A: The powder is the most efficient and the cheapest way to get creatine. However, it is not always convenient, because if you're away somewhere and don't have any supplies around, it can be hard to carry it around and mix it. You can use creatine in any form you prefer, but you have to calculate the dosages. Taking it with a glucose-based product such as fruit juice, especially grape juice, can increase uptake by 10 percent.

I tend to recommend taking creatine with glucose for some of the big athletes who do a lot of lifting. I tell them to take it around the time that they lift, because the glucose seems to help with absorption if they don't get GI (gastrointestinal) stress with it. So they take it about twenty minutes before and after they lift, if they are going to a lengthy lifting session.

Some of the literature suggests that it may be of benefit to take creatine with glycogen supplements, so there are some products on the market that are geared toward replacing glycogen. These can be good for athletes who do both endurance activities and power activities. But taking creatine and glycogen replacement supplements can put stress on the GI system and can cause side effects like bloating, upset stomach, or diarrhea, which people don't want before they work out. So we sometimes suggest grape juice with creatine before and glycogen replacement with creatine after, because we know that glycogen replacements work very effectively after exercise.

Q: Could creatine be helpful for my grandfather, who is in his eighties, not very active, and appears to be getting weaker?

A: Creatine may be beneficial for older adults. We know that it enhances muscle mass and improves fat-free mass in the body. There are a large number of falls and many cases of osteoporosis in the older population, and much of this is due to inadequate muscle strength and co-ordination. That's why an increase in muscle mass may decrease falls, but that is only theoretical at this point.

The real benefit for your grandfather would come if he takes creatine along with a mild resistance-training program. As you know, creatine is far more effective when combined with regular exercise. So whether he does leg lifts in bed, or can work out moderately at home or in a gym, the benefit would be greater. Of course, before he begins taking the creatine or exercis-ing, he would need to consult his physician and work out a program designed for his individual needs. It is also possible that creatine may provide older adults with some cardiovascular benefits as well.

Q: I play high school football and I don't want to use any supplements. But I think that if I don't, I won't be able to compete with everyone else who uses them. What should I do?

A: If you don't want to use any supplements and you believe in doing everything naturally, that is fine. I highly encourage people to stick with natural foods and natural exercise, and I don't think anyone should be pushed or forced to take creatine or other supplements.

Creatine may provide some small benefits in terms of muscle strength and endurance for short-term activities. You need to look at this and weigh its importance for you. I think what is more important is your approach to life. While creatine may provide you with a 10- or 15-percent increase in strength, this may or may not make a difference in your particular sport or activity. And it does not work for everyone. Short-term side effects are minimal, but long-term side effects are unknown.

I recommend that you discuss this situation with your parents and make a decision that is best for you. It's an individual decision that each person needs to make, but only after you have all the available factual information.

Q: I'm a wrestler and I need to keep my weight down. Will I have a problem with gaining weight if I use creatine?

A: You may. Creatine does result in weight gain in most of the people who use it and it could push you out of your weight class as a result.

I'm a former wrestler and I do not recommend creatine in-season for any wrestlers, except heavyweights who do not face any problems with weight gain. There is a limit on heavyweights now, 275 pounds, so if they are not right at the limit, then I recommend that they can take creatine. I do not recommend it to other wrestlers during the season because they need to be very weight conscious in their sport. However, creatine is fine out of season, when they are in the strength-gaining phases of their training program. Keep in mind that they should be off it a minimum of six weeks prior to the beginning of the competitive season and before their weight loss starts.

Q: Is it true that using steroids can make you kill people or commit suicide?

A: We do know that steroids can affect your psychological behavior and this behavior may include severe bouts of anger, which can sometimes be expressed through suicide or murder. But that extreme behavior cannot be solely connected to steroids. It is more likely that the people who commit these acts have some very serious underlying personality problems and that steroids tipped them over the edge into severe anger or poor anger control. This is only one, though possibly the worst, of the dangerous side effects associated with the use of anabolic steroids.

Q: I'm a baseball pitcher and sometimes get involved in very long games that last two or even three hours. Is it a good idea for me to take creatine or any other supplements during the game?

A: I do not recommend taking a creatine supplement during game time. The main benefit of creatine use is to allow you the ability to exercise and recover more quickly. Taking it close to competition time is of little or no benefit and may even pose some performance risks by causing GI distress.

Q: If I decide to cycle, do I load again when I resume taking creatine?

A: That depends on how long you're cycling. If you are off creatine for four to six weeks, you probably should do a loading phase again, because the chances are you're down in your baseline stores. But this varies. Some people can take as long as three months for their levels to drop. It also depends on your cycle period. If you use a short cycle, sometimes you can go with a shorter loading phase or smaller amounts. If you use a longer cycling period, you probably need the full loading phase again.

But it is still not clear what the best way is to go about this. Because what you do also depends on other factors, such as where you are in your training cycle, whether you're in season or out of season, what you are trying to accomplish, what your sport is, or whether you want to avoid rapid weight gain.

Basically, there are four different phases in athletes' programs: preseason, in-season, postseason, and off-season. You need to analyze your specific program and decide if perhaps you want to go through a loading phase in a certain period, then be off creatine during another period. This is highly variable and needs to be worked out with a qualified health-care professional in a plan defining exactly how you are going to use this supplement.

Q: Can you give an example of how creatine might be cycled?

A: I take football players off creatine during the season, so they are not taking it for five months while they are playing. But the team members who are not playing at the time, rehabing or doing other things, are kept on creatine if they so desire. There are many variables.

One of the reasons is that we see a lot of cramping, which may be a result of the creatine, and we don't want that during the playing season. The association with cramping has not yet been scientifically proven, but there was a well-publicized game between Tennessee and Syracuse where many of the Tennessee players came down with cramping. Tennessee was the national champion that year and the next day they blamed creatine for the cramping problem. When they took their players off creatine, there were not as many cramping problems for the rest of the season.

Now, that is not definitive proof. There could be many other explanations for the cramping problem. They were playing inside a dome, they were on turf, it was early in the season, and there were many other factors that could be implicated. There is research going on right now about this and we will have to wait for the results to find out if there is a connection between cramping and creatine use. I personally think that there is a connection.

Q: What if I want to avoid the weight gain of loading?

A: Then you may not want to use a loading phase, because most of the weight gain is within the first week. So you may want to stay with a lower dose and then gradually increase it instead of doing a big loading phase. You need to analyze your individual situation and work out a cohesive plan that you can follow. Whether you load or not, the results should be about the same by the end of one month.

Q: Why don't some people get benefits when they take creatine?

A: There could be a number of reasons. One is that they don't take it on a regular basis and they are not getting enough in. Or maybe they aren't taking the right dose, the amount that their specific body needs. We know that if you take creatine with glucose, it increases the uptake by about 10 percent, so if they do that, it might be effective. Some people may already have high levels of creatine in their muscle and additional amounts are not really going to do anything. Or there may be some genetic factors preventing creatine from working completely in their bodies.

About 20 percent of people who try creatine are non-responders, people who do not see any positive results. If you are one of them, there is no reason to worry about it, but you might discuss it with your health-care professional to see if taking it in a different way might produce results.

Q: I've heard that big muscles from creatine are mostly due to water retention. What is the good of that?

A: A proportion of people using creatine have muscle hypertrophy. This is believed to be a result of three different mechanisms and we are not certain how much is from each mechanism. It is clear that there is water retention within the muscle cell.

However, preliminary research indicates that creatine may improve protein synthesis within the muscle, allowing for enhanced muscle hypertrophy. This research would suggest that the initial gain is from fluid, and then after that it appears to be from some increased protein synthesis and also from the creatine allowing you to recover quicker and therefore train harder.

So these three mechanisms may all play a role: (1) water retention and muscle hypertrophy, (2) protein synthesis, and (3) enhanced training.

Q: I am sixteen and my parents said I can't take creatine because no one knows what could happen down the road. My friends are all taking it and they're fine. How can I convince my parents?

A: I can't advise you to convince your parents. Your parents need to have appropriate information about creatine and they have the right to make ethical decisions about how they want you to use supplements and the value of sports activities. Each decision will be an individual one.

Personally, I cannot encourage younger people to take creatine because I think that people who automatically take it do not understand what they are trying to get out of sports. It's not a matter of being 5 percent better on the bench press. It's a matter of playing, staying healthy, being active, improving your skills, and enjoying the social aspects of being involved in sports. Very few people perform at the highest level in their sport where creatine is going to make a big difference in the performance and outcome of what they are doing.

For example, at a high school level a 5-percent change in bench for an offensive tackle is not going to make a difference in whether he gets a scholarship or not. Far more important is the long-term value for his life, what he got out of sports, whether he learned appropriate social skills, how to interact with colleagues, and the values of exercise, working hard, setting a goal, having discipline, and working as part of a team unit.

To me these things far outweigh everything else. So when parents tell me that they don't want their children using supplements because they are afraid of long-term effects or because they don't want their children buying into the wrong attitude toward sports, I can completely agree with that.

When you're young, it may be hard to understand this. You tend to think that winning and losing are everything and that's what sports are about. So it's good if you can sit down and talk to your parents openly, let your parents clarify their views, find out what they want you to get out of sports, and work along with them for your benefit.

Q: When I took creatine, I got stomach pains and diarrhea the first two days, so I stopped. Does that mean I can never use it?

A: Some people adapt to creatine very well, but a fair amount get gastrointestinal distress with creatine. For those who get GI problems, I would recommend that they skip any large loading phase and instead begin with a small amount and gradually increase it over a period of time.

For example, instead of loading for five to seven days, you should begin with 3 grams of creatine a day and continue on that for perhaps twenty-eight days and see if you adapt to it. If you do not and continue to get an upset stomach, cramps, diarrhea, or other similar problems, these side effects will probably outweigh the benefits you get from creatine, and you will probably be better off without it.

But before you give up completely, try a lower dose, try it with food or different juices, or try reintroducing creatine after being off it for a while and see what happens.

Q: Are you likely to have fewer side effects if you take your creatine with meals instead of between meals?

A: I have not seen that myself. But if you do have problems with creatine, you could try going off it for a few days and then, when you resume, try taking it with something else, which may work for you. Some people who take creatine with a glycogen supplement can get diarrhea, while others will be fine.

You should also look at whether you are getting pure, natural creatine or whether there are other ingredients or contaminants in the creatine you are using. So there are quite a number of things you can do if you have side effects, including checking the quality of your product, taking it with something different, looking at your overall diet, and taking a lower dose.

Q: Is there a real difference between andro and steroids?

A: I don't think there is a real difference. Andro is a precursor and acts at a lower strength. Steroids are banned in sports and andro is readily available in many health-food stores, but we know that the andro pill is probably, in essence, just a reduced version of injectable anabolic steroids.

The other problem is that if you are taking andro, you are very likely to consider using anabolic steroids, even if you believe this is not going to happen. You see results and you feel the push from your peers to take the steroids and before you know it, you give in. Then, it's just a short step to other dangerous drugs. I have seen it happen too many times and it is definitely not worth the risk. So I strongly advise you to stay away from andro altogether.

Q: My husband has Parkinson's disease and is in a wheelchair. Mentally, he is fine, but physically he is very weak. Should I give him creatine?

A: There are studies in the medical journal *Neurology* suggesting that people with neuromuscular problems might be helped by supplementary creatine. Parkinson's is not just a neuromuscular problem, but I would say that people with neuromuscular disorders might benefit from creatine, especially if other aspects of their health are good. But creatine use should be undertaken only with medical supervision and never as a substitute for other medication. You can't go off your regular medications and just take creatine. Talk to your husband's doctor and see if creatine, combined with some physical activity, might be something to try.

Q: I have a friend who is taking all kinds of things, some of them illegal. We are on the college rowing team and I'm afraid something will happen to him. What should I do?

A: Your first step should be to sit down with your

friend and tell him that you are concerned about him and that some of the substances he is taking may be harmful to his health now and in the future. Tell him he should consult a qualified health-care provider for help.

You should also try to understand why your friend may be taking these substances, what belief system he has, what his values are, and what he is trying to get out of his sport. If he does not respond and is unwilling to get medical advice, you could provide him with some information, such as this book, which may be of help.

You should also recognize the fact that if your friend is taking something illegal that is harmful or banned in your sport, and he is on the team, you have an ethical duty to notify someone. College athletes can be drug-tested, and if banned drugs are found, this can lead to disqualification not only for your friend, but for the entire rowing boat. In addition, all your past victories can be wiped out. So your friend is risking not only his own health, but his reputation and that of all his team members and the university as well.

Q: If creatine is found naturally in the body, why didn't nature give us enough for our physical needs? Why do we need supplements?

A: Nature did give us enough for our needs and we do not need supplements. But over time we have continued to push the limits of what our bodies can do. Today, people are bigger, they do more, and they train all year round for their sports. So people's bodies and their physical needs have changed and grown.

We can do fine without creatine or other supplements. But people fall into a mind-set of trying to maximize everything they do, wanting to succeed at the highest level. And sometimes synthetic compounds such as creatine supplements can help.

Creatine has only been available in this country for about ten years, and people have done well throughout the previous years without it. Whether or not to take creatine is an individual decision based on a person's preference and informed decision, not on some innate physical need for additional creatine in order to succeed in sports. Creatine may provide some benefit for certain people and they may want to experiment with taking it. But there is no doubt that you can be successful in sports at the highest levels without it.

Chapter 19

Case Histories

NOTE: The following case histories are composites based on real people who have used creatine and other sports supplements. Their names and identifying factors have been changed in order to protect their privacy.

BRIAN: BUILDING SIZE FOR COLLEGE FOOTBALL

When eighteen-year-old Brian entered college as a freshman, he was six feet two inches tall and weighed 210 pounds. Although that may sound big to some, he found that in his first year the other football players he was competing with were older, more muscular, and weighed more, on average about 230 pounds. As a result Brian had difficulty with certain plays because he did not have the size, strength, or endurance of some of the other players.

Brian consulted Dr. Monaco about what he could do to gain more muscle mass, strength, and stamina. Dr. Monaco asked him many questions about his eating, exercise, and lifestyle. He found that Brian often skipped meals and ate a diet high in fat. He had also tried many different vitamins and shakes in an attempt to improve his strength and endurance.

Dr. Monaco and Brian talked about his health, diet, and the possible use of creatine monohydrate or other supplements. Brian talked about why he wanted to use creatine and what he hoped to achieve from it. Dr. Monaco pointed out that although creatine appears to be safe at this time, there is no information available about long-term use, so there is some risk in using it. Together they worked out a program to improve Brian's athletic potential. In addition Dr. Monaco encouraged Brian to discuss his concerns with his family and keep them informed about what he was doing.

At the end of Brian's freshman football season Dr. Monaco placed him on an aggressive weight-training program in order to build up his muscle mass. Brian lifted weights four to five times a week and tried to eat a diet high in calories and protein in order to increase his weight.

Dr. Monaco also referred Brian to a nutritionist for additional help with his diet. Under the nutritionist's guidance Brian started to take creatine with grape juice at the loading dose of 5 grams four times a day, which he did for five days. He then switched to the maintenance dose of 3 grams with grape juice twice a day. He reported no adverse side effects from the creatine.

After only ten days on the nutrition and exercise program, Brian saw an immediate weight gain of five pounds. He also found that he had greater stamina toward the end of his lengthy weight-training workouts.

"I can do much more work at the end of my lifting sessions," he commented, "and I don't get tired the way I used to." Over the next two months Brian's strength trainers also noted a marked increase in his strength. By the start of his sophomore year Brian's weight had increased to 235 pounds and his strength on key exercises was significantly greater. As a result he can compete far more effectively with the other football players and expects to see much more playing time with his college team.

HANNAH: AN AVID TRIATHLETE

Training vigorously five days a week, thirty-two-year-old Hannah is a dedicated triathlete who supplements her diets with numerous vitamins. She has recently started taking creatine.

But Hannah is concerned because she is thinking about getting pregnant in the next two years and she wants to be certain that there are no problems with her taking creatine. So Hannah consulted Dr. Monaco.

In discussing creatine with Hannah, Dr. Monaco explained that there is limited research on the long-term risks of creatine and there is no research on its effects on pregnancy. Although creatine is made naturally in the body and, if taken in its pure form as a supplement, should not pose a problem, Dr. Monaco explained that there are still theoretical risks to her unborn baby.

"I am stopping the creatine for now," explained Hannah, "just to be safe. I don't want to take any chances.

After the baby I might try it again." In addition Dr. Monaco also advised Hannah to remain on a healthy diet and take her essential vitamins, as she continues to train prior to becoming pregnant.

MIKE: CREATINE FOR BASKETBALL?

Nineteen years old and a starting point guard on the college basketball team, Mike recently heard that some pro basketball players are using creatine and he was naturally curious about whether it might be helpful for him.

"I've never tried any supplements before," Mike explained, "because I like doing everything naturally. But everyone on the team is taking it, so maybe I should take it too. That is, if it's safe."

Encouraged by his coach to get more information, Mike went to both his strength coach and Dr. Monaco for some guidance.

Dr. Monaco explained what creatine is and that it is a natural substance in the body. However, he also told Mike that creatine primarily benefits athletes in power sports such as football, throwing events, and sprints, where it can help increase weight and strength needed for short repetitive exercise. At this time the scientific literature does not support creatine's benefits for basketball, added Dr. Monaco.

Despite the fact that everyone on the team seemed to be using it, Mike was relieved to hear that he didn't really need creatine. Placed on a sound nutritional diet and encouraged to work hard in all aspects of his sport, Mike is doing well enough at basketball to compete at the highest level.

JOE: CONCERNED ABOUT DRUG TESTS

"I've been taking creatine for the past few months," Joe told Dr. Monaco, "but I'm not sure it's helping me."

A twenty-one-year-old college football player, Joe consulted Dr. Monaco because his university, for legal and ethical reasons, does not recommend creatine, and he was taking it on his own because he felt he needed any advantage he could get. Joe also felt he did not know enough about what he was doing.

"This stuff is so expensive, so I just buy the cheapest one or whatever is on sale," Joe told Dr. Monaco. "I've used quite a few different brands and I've tried different creatine powders, liquids, and pills. I can't tell if it's helping me and I'm also worried that it may show up on some drug test and I'll be in trouble."

In addition Joe wanted to find out how long it would take to get the creatine out of his system and if he should stop using it right away because of the drug tests. Joe said that his university suspends for up to a year players they find "positive" on their drug tests during which time they are not allowed to participate in their sport.

Dr. Monaco asked Joe if he was using any other supplements or drugs, and Joe said he wasn't. He said he drank beer occasionally, but that was all. Then, Dr. Monaco told Joe how creatine is made naturally in the body and is not banned by the NCAA, is not classified as a drug, and cannot be detected in any current drug testing and, in fact, is not even tested for to begin with.

He informed Joe that it takes between two and six weeks for supplemental creatine to clear the body entirely, depending on the individual's size and other dosing issues.

Dr. Monaco also pointed out to Joe that by taking so many different products, he is not certain what he is actually taking at any given time. Some of these products may be pure creatine, while others may be mixed with other ingredients, including some, like ephedrine, which *are* banned by some sports governing institutions.

Joe was advised to read the labels carefully to make sure the creatine supplement he uses does not contain any banned substances. Dr. Monaco pointed out that if Joe tests positive on a drug test because he is taking some banned substance, his ignorance that the substance was in his supplement will not be an acceptable excuse. Joe, in fact, is responsible for everything he puts in his body and he must read the labels and know what he is doing.

So if Joe wants to continue using creatine, he should buy the same product all the time, one from a well-established, reputable company. Dr. Monaco offered to check the product for Joe and even to send it out to a lab for analysis, if Joe felt it was necessary.

Following this advice, Joe decided to continue taking creatine for the time being. He purchased a product that was pure creatine, with no other ingredients and produced by a well-known, recommended company, and he also checked his doses very carefully.

JOHN: A RECREATIONAL
WEIGHT LIFTER

Forty-two years old, John enjoys physical activity and is very health conscious. He weighs 180 pounds and is five feet ten inches tall, with a lean, muscular body. Although he lifts weights three times a week and is very serious about his sport, John is a recreational athlete, is not involved in bodybuilding, and does not enter competitions. He also jogs about five miles twice a week to stay in shape.

In his weight-lifting sessions John works out for about an hour, gearing his activities toward high repetitions and endurance. He keeps up with the sports literature and is always looking for ways to improve his skills and results. So when John heard about Mark McGwire and his use of creatine, he was immediately interested. He consulted Dr. Monaco for more information, hoping to find out if creatine might be a good supplement for his needs, although he added that he had some concerns about possible side effects.

John told Dr. Monaco that he was concerned because as he got older, it was harder for him to see gains in his strength. He wondered if perhaps creatine might provide that extra boost that would help him.

Dr. Monaco explained that creatine works naturally in the body and helps with anaerobic activities, such as weight lifting. He told John that creatine can help some people gain weight and improve their strength for short-term power activities, especially those that involve multiple repetitions lasting under ten seconds. Creatine, Dr. Monaco told John, can even provide significant gains for certain people at the highest levels of their sport where tenths of a second can be the difference in placing in a competition.

But since John is a recreational athlete and is not involved in high-level competitions or the training that would be involved, Dr. Monaco concluded that if John decided to use creatine, he would probably experience only a slight improvement in his performance and it would not make a significant difference for him.

Finally, since John is very concerned about good health and tries to follow a beneficial program, creatine might not be a good choice because of the unknown long-term health risks it might pose.

"I learned a lot about creatine," commented John, "and decided that I wasn't going to take it. I didn't want to find out a few years down the line that it had some dangerous side effects." Since John did not see any major benefits in using creatine, either for his sports performance or his health, he continued his exercise program without adding creatine.

MANNY: TRAINING ISSUES

A wrestler in the 125-pound group, Manny has read a great deal about creatine and has also talked to many health-care professionals about it.

"I know that creatine is not good for wrestlers during the season," he explained, "but I also do weight lifting in the summer and I want to get into the 140-pound wrestling class by next year. So I need to gain some weight."

So with hopes of making the 140-pound class by

building up his muscle mass, Manny consulted Dr. Monaco to find out if creatine might help him in his off-season.

Dr. Monaco talked with Manny, explaining that even though creatine may not be useful during the wrestling season, that does not mean it can't be helpful in off-season. He explained the concept of periodization, meaning that an athlete's season should be broken down into four basic phases: preseason, in-season, post-season, and off-season.

Each of these four phases has different requirements. For Manny creatine could be a viable option during his off-season and could help him to build up strength and weight.

After discussing all the risks and benefits of using creatine, Manny decided to try creatine during the summer and report back to Dr. Monaco if he experienced any problems with it. He will stop using it at least six weeks before the wrestling season begins and will see if the creatine, along with his exercise and diet program, will help him reach his goals.

HAROLD: ELDERLY AND WORN OUT

When Harold's daughter brought him to see Dr. Monaco, he was seventy-eight years old, not physically active, and experiencing increasing problems with fatigue and getting out of chairs. She was concerned about her father's health and was looking for some way to improve his situation.

"I have a good appetite," Harold told the doctor, "and I'm pretty healthy. I've never had any problems with my kidneys, liver, muscles, bones, or anything. But I'm feel-

ing very weak lately and I don't like it." Harold added
that he was very interested in supplements and had read
about creatine and DHEA.

Dr. Monaco gave Harold a complete physical examination and full blood chemistry tests to check for baseline functioning of his liver, kidneys, and thyroid gland.
He also had a urinalysis. When all of Harold's tests
checked out normal, Dr. Monaco recommended that
Harold begin a generalized strength-and-balance training program to help reduce the chances of a fall and possibly a hip fracture, which is so common in older people.

Dr. Monaco explained the potential benefits of using
creatine to enhance Harold's short-term strength for
anaerobic activities.

"I've never taken any supplements before," Harold
commented, "but this one sounds pretty safe and my
daughter thinks I should try it. So I'm leaning that way."

If he does decide to use creatine and follow the exercise program, Harold could gain some benefits in
strength and stamina.

JACK: WHICH TYPE TO USE?

"I've used creatine for the past two years," said Jack,
a twenty-six-year-old avid bodybuilder who lifts six
times a week. "And I've seen real improvements in my
strength and endurance during lifting sessions."

Jack is six feet four inches tall, weighs 240 pounds,
and says he has gained seven pounds since he started
using creatine. He credits the supplement with providing him additional energy toward the end of his lengthy
lifting sessions.

Jack's problem is choosing the best form of creatine for his needs. Since he works out in the gym six days a week, he finds it difficult to bring powdered creatine there and mix it. So he has been taking 3 grams of the powder in the morning and another 3 grams before bed. But he doesn't feel that these are the best times to take it and he wonders if pills or premixed creatine drinks might be better.

Jack came to Dr. Monaco and discussed his concerns. Dr. Monaco explained that so far, no studies have proven that any one form of creatine (powder, liquid, gel, pills) is superior to any other form. But he did tell Jack that he has to be sure that he is getting the right dose.

Because of the amount Jack takes, he might have to swallow as many as ten pills at a time, which is more trouble for him than mixing up a powder drink in the morning. He also understands the benefit of taking creatine with a glucose drink.

In addition to the question of what form to use, Dr. Monaco also discussed the benefits of stopping creatine altogether for a while, perhaps every few months or when his training schedule is reduced. Since we don't know the long-term effects yet, taking a break every few months could be a way of protecting yourself in case side effects are discovered down the road.

After this consultation Jack decided to continue with the creatine powder in the morning and evening, and to cycle creatine, with periodic breaks every few months, because of safety concerns.

THOMAS: ELEVEN
AND UNDERWEIGHT

A Pop Warner/midget football player, Thomas is eleven years old, but is very small for his age and is under the minimum weight for football in his town. Thomas's dad is a former college football player and is naturally very eager to see his son play the game. He has been giving Thomas weight-gain shakes and drinks, but Thomas is still five pounds below the minimum. Would creatine be helpful for him?

Thomas's dad asked his son's pediatrician for advice, and he referred them to Dr. Monaco.

First, Dr. Monaco explained that although creatine could help people put on weight, often about five pounds, it is not well studied in children and could present a risk. Then, Dr. Monaco engaged Thomas's father in a discussion about his views on sports for young children.

"I had a great time playing football when I was young," the father told Dr. Monaco, "and of course I want the same thing for Thomas. It's only a matter of a few pounds, so there should be some way to help him gain it."

Dr. Monaco explained that for children, it's best for sports to be enjoyable and an activity that can help them improve their physical health, develop beneficial lifestyle patterns, and promote psychological well-being. If Thomas learns to interact well with other children, participate in teamwork, accept both winning and losing, and understand how to set goals, he will get a lot out of sports, even if he is not always the most outstanding member of his team.

Using supplements at such a young age, Dr. Monaco noted, could really take the focus off what should be the important aspects of sports and put the stress solely on the competitive aspect.

In consultation with Dr. Monaco, Thomas, his father, and his mother all agree that he should be able to gain weight, perhaps more slowly, but more naturally, by following a supervised strength-training program and a good diet. Eventually his body will mature and he will gain the weight naturally and be able to qualify for the team, if that is what he really wants to do.

CHARLES: LOU GEHRIG'S DISEASE

Barely able to move on his own, Charles is a thirty-nine-year-old man suffering from Lou Gehrig's disease (also known as ALS), a neuromuscular condition. Charles has full nursing care and no other medical problems.

After reading about a recent study reported in the journal *Neurology*, Charles wanted to get more information about creatine. The study showed that using creatine supplements appeared to be more effective than the medication he was using, in helping patients to regain some muscular strength.

After consulting by phone with Dr. Monaco, Charles was told that this was only one study and it used a very small number of patients, although the results are quite hopeful. He was informed about the possible risks, as well as the benefits, of supplemental creatine.

"If it helped them, it might be able to help me too,"

said Charles. So Dr. Monaco recommended that Charles consider a trial period of creatine under the supervision of his neurologist. After two months Charles finds that he has gained some weight and strength. He is happy with the results and is continuing to use creatine for his health condition.

KELLY: A COMPETITIVE CYCLIST

Twenty-four-year-old Kelly is a recreational cyclist, but she also participates in summer road competitions. Kelly loves riding and also loves winning and trains very hard in her sport.

"A lot of cyclists are taking creatine and all other kinds of supplements," commented Kelly, "and I don't take anything. Am I missing something?"

Kelly went to see Dr. Monaco to get his advice. He asked her if the cyclists who are taking creatine have had any positive benefits.

"I don't know," Kelly told him. "I know some of them didn't see any improvements, so they stopped. I'm not sure about the others. It's hard to tell."

Dr. Monaco explained that even though creatine is a natural substance found in the body, it could prove to be harmful if taken long-term. We just aren't sure as yet. He noted also that there have been very few studies on the use of creatine with women, especially in terms of how it might affect the menstrual cycle or other aspects of the female body. In addition, creatine has not been shown to be of benefit in aerobic activities, such as distance cycling, so it is unlikely that Kelly would benefit from it anyway.

But Dr. Monaco also told her that for repeated six- to thirty-second bouts of maximal stationary cycling, with recovery periods of twenty seconds to five minutes, creatine can be an ergogenic aid. However, this has only been demonstrated in a lab study under controlled conditions and may not pertain to the kinds of events that Kelly participates in.

"I don't think I'm going to use creatine," Kelly concluded. "It doesn't sound like it would do anything for my sport and it will be one less thing to think about."

JOSH: WHAT DOSE TO TAKE?

Starting on creatine in high school at the recommendation of his friends and lifting buddies at the gym, Josh took the supplement on and off. He did not discuss it with his parents, using his allowance to pay for his supplies. But because of the cost, Josh did not take the supplement on a regular basis.

"I took the creatine about four times a week, when I did weight lifting," explained Josh. "I didn't do loading and missed a lot of days and sometimes went off it for a few weeks. I didn't see much difference in my performance, but it seemed to help a lot of my friends who took it every day."

When he went to college and started playing football, Josh consulted Dr. Monaco about possibly using creatine on a regular basis in order to build up his weight and strength. Dr. Monaco told Josh about the pros and cons of creatine use and that if he wanted to use it, he would have to make a commitment to use it properly.

Josh decided to use a loading dose of 5 grams of creatine four times a day for five days, then a maintenance dose of 3 grams a day with grape juice twice a day. After a trial of six weeks in the off-season, combined with regular workouts, John found that he had gained three pounds and increased muscle size. He reported that he had not missed any doses and was very pleased with the results.

STEVE: PROBLEMS WITH AIDS

Steve has had AIDS-related health problems for the past seven years, and has been hospitalized several times for different infections, including pneumonia. Thirty-two years old, Steve takes many AIDS medications and has lost a great deal of weight over the past five years.

"I was 130 pounds when I was healthy," said Steve, who is five feet three inches tall, "and now I'm only 110. I never seem to have much of an appetite and don't eat a lot, even though I try. I feel pretty weak most of the time."

Steve's doctor consulted Dr. Monaco to see if creatine might be helpful for him in terms of weight gain and building up his physical strength. He was told that Steve had tried several alternative therapies in an effort to build up his body, but nothing had helped. As a result of his disease Steve's muscles are in a state of severe wasting and he has had to cut back drastically on his activities.

Dr. Monaco explained that recent studies indicate that creatine may be of benefit to people with muscle wasting and other neuromuscular diseases. He said that because of Steve's condition, it might be worthwhile to give creatine a try, even though the long-term effects remain unknown. When compared to some of the medications Steve is using, creatine is relatively safe.

Dr. Monaco placed Steve on creatine after cautioning him that his progress had to be closely monitored to be certain there is no adverse effect on his kidneys and no side effects from combining creatine with his different medications.

For Steve creatine is a success story. After only two weeks, he reported to Dr. Monaco, "I've gained six pounds, the first weight I've gained in years. I feel stronger, even though I still can't do a lot, but I hope I will gain more strength as I continue taking it." Steve did not experience any adverse side effects and said that he plans to continue taking creatine, along with his medications, in the hope that he will see even more improvement in the weeks and months ahead.

KEN: SIDE EFFECTS

"I never had a problem with creatine back home," explained Ken, a twenty-year-old college football player. "This cramping is very strange."

But there is a possible explanation.

Ken comes from a northern part of the United States and is now a college student in the South. He plays football and takes creatine with at least one glass of water. He reported no health problems and appeared to be in good physical shape when he joined the team.

The university medical staff found his preliminary blood work normal. He was informed about the benefits and risks of creatine, the lack of information on long-term effects, and the potential for kidney stress. Ken was also advised to stop taking creatine during the twice-a-day practices of football camp and to increase his water intake to prevent dehydration and reduce kidney stress. Finally, he was told that creatine takes between two and six weeks to clear his system.

Following this advice, Ken stopped taking creatine and began to drink large amounts of water during the football camp. But one day Ken experienced a severe episode of muscle cramps in his hamstrings, forcing him to miss an entire day of training.

Ken's doctor told him that these cramps could possibly be associated with creatine use, although nothing can be proven. There are many reports of muscle cramping with athletes on creatine. But the doctor also points out that Ken is now in a hot, humid climate and he is performing more activity than he did in the past, so those factors could also have contributed to his cramping.

Ken's doctor monitors him for further cramping, which does not occur, and Ken stays off creatine until the off-season, which seems a good solution.

SALVATORE: HEALTH PROBLEMS

A recreational athlete and power lifter, thirty-two-year-old Salvatore has also had a number of health problems, including nephrotic syndrome, a kidney disorder. Salvatore sees his doctor regularly and is on a low-protein diet.

Thinking that creatine might help him to improve his bench press and clean and jerk, Salvatore developed an interest in the supplement. His power-lifter friends told him that creatine gave them good results, but Salvatore is worried about the effect that creatine might have on his kidneys.

Consulting Dr. Monaco, Salvatore is told that creatine is cleared by the kidneys and therefore could possibly present an increased stress, which would not be good for him. However, Dr. Monaco also explained that studies have not been done for more than a two-year period and so far, no detrimental effects by creatine on the kidneys have been proven.

But there is another problem that could affect Salvatore. When people take creatine, its presence can affect the results of certain blood tests that doctors perform to test kidney function. Because of that it is possible that a patient may have misleading test results due to the supplement.

Understanding these problems, Salvatore agreed when Dr. Monaco advised him that because of his history of kidney disease, it would not be a good idea for him to use creatine.

"I know that creatine might have helped my lifting a little, but I'd rather be safe, so I'm not going to take it," Salvatore concluded.

EUGENE: GETTING INFORMATION

A seventeen-year-old resident of rural Arkansas, Eugene has heard about creatine and read about it on the Internet. Curious about whether it might benefit him, Eugene consulted his doctor, but the doctor didn't know much about it and couldn't really advise him.

Eugene turned to his parents for help, but they didn't know anything about creatine, so together they decided to try to get some reliable information.

The athletic trainer at Eugene's school offered to call a doctor he knew, who said that Eugene should check at the local university and talk to the team physician. He also suggested that he contact the state medical school to see if any of their doctors have a special interest in creatine or sports supplements. Usually, sports-medicine physicians will have this knowledge.

Finally, Eugene was advised to try the Internet, including Web sites like www.sportsci.org, which has scientific reviews of supplements, including creatine.

Eugene and his parents followed this advice and were able to get reliable information on creatine from the Internet and from a sports physician at the nearest university. Since Eugene was seventeen, a basketball player, and a healthy, well-built, strong young man, they all agreed that creatine would probably not be worth the time or expense. In the future, if Eugene becomes intensely involved in anaerobic sports in college, they can reevaluate the situation.

BRUCE: COLLEGE SPRINTER

"My friends who throw the shot put and discus are all using creatine and they tell me it really helps," said Bruce, a nineteen-year-old college sprinter. Bruce's times in his sprints are very good and he is just a fraction of a second from making qualifiers for the regional competitions.

Bruce consulted Dr. Monaco about whether or not he

should try creatine and if it might provide him with the boost to help him to qualify.

Dr. Monaco discussed many issues with Bruce, including the possible benefits and the possible downside of his trying creatine. He explained that scientific studies on a single bout of sprinting with creatine are inconclusive, some studies indicating it can help and others that it could actually hurt performance. There is also no conclusive evidence on whether creatine is helpful for repetitive sprints.

In addition, Bruce could gain weight on creatine, which might be a problem for him as a sprinter, since it could actually slow him down.

Considering all this information, Bruce decided not to use creatine for the time being and to try to keep informed about future studies to see if some proven benefits for sprinters might turn up. He is also considering the possibility of trying it over the summer when there is less pressure on him.

MICHAEL: WHAT TO TELL MY PARENTS

On the thin side, fifteen-year-old Michael participates in several different sports, including baseball in the spring and soccer in the winter. He also likes to lift weights for fun a few days a week.

Michael is thinking about using creatine to try to build up his physique. "I'm tired of being thin," he explained, "and I want to put on some bulk."

During his annual physical exam for sports, Michael asked Dr. Monaco if there are any supplements that could help him. Dr. Monaco talked with Michael about the positive and negative aspects of creatine and encouraged him to discuss this with his parents. Michael responded that he wasn't very comfortable discussing these things with his parents, but that he would give it a try.

That evening, when his parents asked about his exam, Michael told them what Dr. Monaco had said about creatine. His parents seemed surprised and asked him why he would want to take a supplement and what he expected to get from it. They pointed out that many supplements are heavily publicized, with lots of claims for their benefits, and they just don't pan out and eventually disappear.

Michael's parents impressed on him their conviction that excellence in sports is about far more than just taking a pill or a supplement and some of these substances, like tryptophan and ephedrine, have been proven to be harmful.

Finally, his parents pointed out that even if creatine improved his strength, Michael's benefits from his sports activities would not be that different.

"I decided not to use creatine," Michael said, "because I don't think I really need it. I've improved my diet and I'm training more and making progress and I think I'm happy the way I am."

MARK: A DANGER TO WRESTLERS?

A wrestler in the 190-pound class, Mark naturally weighs about 188 pounds and he lifts during the season. In the past he wanted to take creatine, but his coach and parents warned him not to use it because they had heard about the deaths of three wrestlers who used creatine.

"I didn't really believe it," noted Mark. "Lots of my sports friends were taking creatine and they seemed fine. If it could kill you, I don't think the government would let people buy it. It would be banned."

To find out the real story Mark asked Dr. Monaco for his advice.

Dr. Monaco explained that the three wrestlers who died did not die as a result of using creatine. Rather, it was a result of excessive weight loss, as much as fifteen pounds in a short period of time, which caused dehydration and kidney malfunction. Inside the body toxic chemicals built up and eventually caused the heart to stop beating.

Some people who use creatine can become dehydrated, Dr. Monaco told Mark, and it is important to take it with a lot of fluids. In addition, creatine is not recommended for wrestlers during the season, or for wrestlers who need to lose weight, which should always be done gradually.

However, for wrestlers in the upper weight classes, creatine can play a part if used properly. Since wrestling is an anaerobic activity, wrestlers who are not concerned about weight gain and who remain hydrated may benefit from creatine supplementation during their off-season.

Armed with the correct information, Mark decided that he would like to give it a try. He now plans to use creatine for a few weeks during the off-season to see the effects and he will check back with Dr. Monaco prior to the beginning of the wrestling season.

Dr. Monaco also gave Mark an information packet that he can share with his parents so they will also be fully informed on the benefits and risks of using supplemental creatine.

Chapter 20

A Final Word

By now you have learned a great deal about creatine and other natural muscle-enhancing supplements. Perhaps you wanted this information in order to help you decide whether or not you should use them. Perhaps you are already taking some of these supplements and want to find out how they work, whether they are safe, and which ones are right for your individual needs. Or perhaps you are a parent and are concerned about your children using supplements.

There are no simple or easy answers to the question "Should I use creatine or other natural supplements to help me with my sports performance?" You have seen how many different factors and issues can come into play, and each person must come up with an individual answer.

But there are a number of important points that you should keep in mind as you try to make the decision that will work best for you.

DO NOT MAKE YOUR DECISION ALONE

No matter how old you are, how informed you are, or how experienced you are in life, you should not make your decision about using supplements by yourself.

Everyone who considers using supplements should consult a physician first and discuss the situation in detail. You should have a thorough medical checkup and any tests your doctor feels are necessary.

If possible, you will want to see a physician who is familiar with creatine and other sports supplements. If you can't find a doctor with these qualifications, you should ask your doctor to read the literature prior to your visit.

Other people you may want to consult are your coach, trainer, and nutritionist. Chances are, they will be well informed about sports supplements and will be able to give you some guidance.

If you are still a student, you should definitely talk about supplement use with your parents. Again, if they are not familiar with these substances, you should provide them with some reading material before you talk.

Finally, you can also listen to the experiences of your friends and acquaintances who have been using supplements. But when you do this, you should remember that everyone is different and just because one of your teammates had what he describes as "great results" with some supplement, that does not mean it is also right for you.

So while you want to collect information from the

people you know, you should never base your decision on whether to use supplements on the experiences of your friends.

BE CONSERVATIVE

If you decide that you want to try supplements, and you feel you have good reasons for doing so, do not get carried away. Don't rush to the health-food store and buy everything in sight and rush home to take it.

Instead, begin with one supplement. According to everything we know, creatine is definitely one of the safer and better choices for anaerobic sports, provided you fit the criteria that we have outlined.

Recent research indicates that you can do just as well with a regular dose as you can with a loading period, it just takes longer. So if you do not want to begin with larger amounts and have no compelling reason to do so, it is fine to start with a regular dose of between 2 and 4 grams a day, or the appropriate dose for your size.

If you are consistent in your use and have patience, you should see results within a few weeks. Remember that we do not know the long-term effects of creatine use, so if you take a low dose and you cycle, with periods of weeks or months when you do not use it, you will probably be safer, at least until more research is available.

MAINTAIN MEDICAL SUPERVISION

When you use creatine or any other sports supplements, it is important that your doctor or other health-care professional see you regularly to monitor you for any adverse effects.

In addition, if you experience any side effects, you should immediately report them and follow your doctor's advice about what to do, whether it is to take a lower dose, take your supplements in some other way, or stop them altogether.

You should also have any periodic medical tests that your doctor recommends in order to monitor your physical health. Not all changes in the body are apparent and sometimes tests can be useful warnings that something is not right.

STAY INFORMED

Since creatine and the other sports supplements we have discussed are not prescription medications and are not approved by the FDA, they have not been as rigorously tested. Long-term studies are in progress, but the results are not yet available. In addition, many other studies are ongoing and it is important to keep up-to-date as their findings are released.

New information can be found in many daily newspapers, weekly magazines and sports publications, and online at various sports and nutritional-supplement sites.

In addition, many health-food stores have well-informed personnel who can help you keep updated on the latest information about these supplements. If you are really serious about your data, you can also consult the nearest public medical library and read the actual studies as they are published in the journals.

Although many years of studies have indicated that creatine is very safe, especially for short-term use, there is no way to predict what future studies may uncover.

WEIGH THE BENEFITS
AND THE RISKS

It is easy to get carried away by the latest craze, and creatine certainly qualifies as a major supplement phenomenon.

But as you have seen, it is not necessarily a good supplement for everyone. You will have to determine yourself whether it might be helpful and safe for you.

One way you can do that is to weigh the different benefits and risks that apply to you. Many people find it helpful to write these down and compare them.

You can divide a page in half and on the left side put down all the benefits you think you can get from taking creatine. On the right side put down your potential risks if you use this supplement. Then take a good look at your lists and see which side is stronger.

Your "risk" side can include any negative factors, such as the cost and the inconvenience of taking a supplement. Of course, you will also consider the specific types of exercise and sports you engage in and whether creatine has been shown to be effective for those activities.

DON'T EXPECT MIRACLES

If you make the decision to use creatine or any other supplement, do not expect stunning, overnight changes. You will not go from being a 90-pound weakling to being a 220-pound monster, no matter how much creatine you take.

At best creatine helps about 80 percent of the people who use it and makes a difference in performance of between 10 and 15 percent. But the gains you experience will all be the result of the hard physical work that goes along with your supplement, not the substance alone.

Think of creatine as a possible helper on your road to sports excellence. It may give you a small boost, but it is really the hard work you put in that makes the difference.

REMEMBER WHAT SPORTS IS ALL ABOUT

Do not allow yourself to get carried away by the need to always be the best, to win at all costs, and to do anything and everything to achieve that goal.

Yes, it is wonderful to win an Olympic gold medal, and if an athlete was not single-minded in that pursuit, the goal would probably never be achieved. But winning an Olympic medal is only for the very few, and most athletes do not have that goal.

For most people involved in sports, there are other goals, including the pure physical enjoyment of playing, being part of a team, sharing goals and helping one another, feeling good, and improving your health.

Moderation in all things is a useful motto and one that will remind you not to get too focused on sports competition. Of course, you will always try to do your best and you will work hard to maximize your potential. But life is more than just competitive sports.

Creatine has a place in the world of sports nutrition. It is up to you to find out if it has a place in your world and, if so, what that place will be. If you make your decisions carefully, whether they are to use it or not, your chances of good results are quite high.

Index